MY BABY'S BOOK OF CHILD HEALTH

THE INFANT AND TODDLER YEARS

Crane Publishing Company, Inc.

Complete Contents Copyright © 1969
by Crane Publishing Company, Inc.

All Rights Reserved

Printed in the United States of America

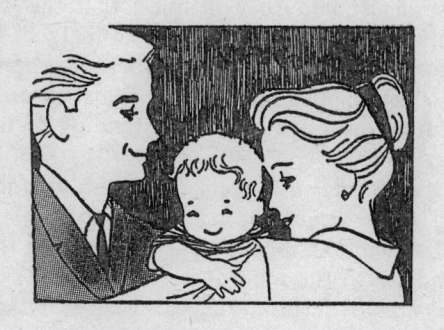

Introduction to
MY BABY's Book Of Child Health

OVER the course of the years, MY BABY Magazine and its affiliated publications have printed many excellent original articles on pregnancy, infant care and training by competent medical authorities. Unless the reader clips his reading material for filing purposes or has the mind of a computer, these contributions are doomed to oblivion. Therefore, the staff of MY BABY has selected what they consider the best and most practical of more than 200 articles by physicians published by Crane Publications, and created this important anthology, MY BABY'S BOOK OF CHILD HEALTH.

The reader should keep in mind that this book is not a substitute for a good doctor. The material in it is intended to bring a mother or a mother-to-be up-to-date with the latest happenings in the fields covered and make her more receptive and understanding of medical advice given her.

As an obstetrician, I realize how important good health and sound health principals are to the strength of the next generation. The more that is learned through research and study, the more it is realized that even before the process of fertilization, the health and genetic normalcy of the potential parents play a significant role. Youth, good nutrition, sound health and normal chromosomes each play a powerful part. After pregnancy and delivery the diet of the infant and the young child is extremely important, as proved by the mental damage done by protein deficiency in the early critical years. Then, too, the importance of intellectual stimulation in the cradle and stroller has been brought home to us by the cruel mental handicaps suffered by neglected children.

I hope that you, the reader, will read MY BABY'S BOOK OF CHILD HEALTH from cover to cover. I feel sure you will get much value from it, as well as hours pleasantly spent.

Alan F. Guttmacher, M.D.
President, Planned Parenthood Federation of America, Inc.

Publisher's Note

Readers of MY BABY Magazine have, for many years, had the advice and opinions of many of the leading doctors in the country in solving their pregnancy and baby care problems. Thousands of them have responded to this sage counsel by writing to the various doctors for help with their own personal problems. Rarely, if ever, have their letters gone unanswered.

Because of our readers' obviously deep interest in these medical articles, we decided to put as many of them as possible into book form. This compact little book contains much valuable and helpful information pertaining to those vital subjects that mothers and mothers-to-be want to know more about. Each doctor represented here is an authority on the subject on which he has written; his point of view has a special value because it is in practical, everyday use and is not merely theory.

The question of each doctor's own point of view brings up another interesting detail. Doctors—like people —like all of us—are different. Three pediatricians may have three different attitudes toward the same problem of baby care. These differences are to be expected. They do not signify that anyone of the three doctors is wrong; they simply indicate that each doctor has found his own particular solution most efficacious and practical with his patients.

Naturally, our readers will have their own doctor's counsel and advice which will, in the last analysis, be the advice they will follow. Yet there are wise words and recommendations here which will be very helpful to every mother who reads this book.

Because of these differing medical opinions, and because each doctor represented here is an individualist with a definite philosophy on his own special subject, we must place all responsibility for opinions and statements in these articles on the doctor's own shoulders. After all, that is the way he would want it.

Willard L. Crane
Publisher

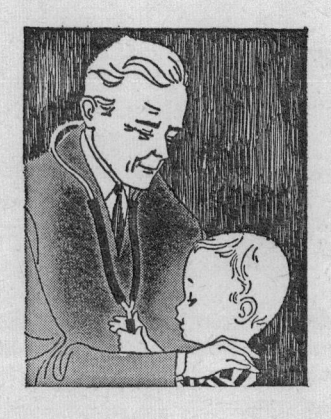

TABLE OF CONTENTS

Foreword—Alan F. Guttmacher, M.D.	3
Publisher's Note—Willard L. Crane	5
Contributing Doctors	11
SECTION I—Preparing For The Baby	13
Diet and Weight Control in Pregnancy—by Alan F. Guttmacher, M.D.	14
Nutrition and Childbirth—by Elizabeth D. Munves, Ph.D.	19
Minor Complaints of Pregnancy—by Alan F. Guttmacher, M.D.	23
Dental Care For The Expectant Mother—by Harold Sherman, D.D.S.	30
For a Healthy Pregnancy—by Alan F. Guttmacher, M.D.	34
Care of the Feet During Pregnancy—by Morton H. Walker, D.S.C.	39
Management of Twin Pregnancy—by Alan F. Guttmacher, M.D.	42
Rh (Erythroblastosis)—by R. Cannon Eley, M.D.	45
The Father's Role—by Alan F. Guttmacher, M.D.	48
Advice to New Mothers—by Alan F. Guttmacher, M.D.	52

TABLE OF CONTENTS

SECTION II—Caring For The Newborn 54

The New Arrival—by Alfred J. Vignec, M.D. 55

Diaper Rash—by R. Cannon Eley, M.D. 60

Care of Baby's Skin—by H. Laurence Dowd, M.D. ... 63

The Art of Mothering—by Dorothy V. Whipple, M.D. 66

At Home With Baby—by Herbert M. Porter, M.D. ... 69

Sound Sleep Habits—by Dorothy V. Whipple, M.D. 73

Colic and the Nervous Baby—by Helen Evans Reid, M.D. 76

Making a Feeding Schedule—by Alfred J. Vignec, M.D. 80

The Premature Baby—by R. Cannon Eley, M.D. 85

PKU (Phenylketonuria)—by R. Cannon Eley, M.D. 88

SECTION III—As The Baby Grows 92

Common Infections—by R. Cannon Eley, M.D. 93

Colds—by Dorothy V. Whipple, M.D. 97

Keep Him Creeping—by Melvin Schrier, O.D. 102

Toilet Training—by Alfred J. Vignec, M.D. 106

Your Baby's Sight—by Melvin Schrier, O.D. 113

Your Child's Feet—by Morton H. Walker, D.S.C. 116

Immunization Chart—by Frank Howard Richardson, M.D. 122

TABLE OF CONTENTS

SECTION IV—Feeding and Nutrition 124

Modern Feeding Practices—by Elizabeth D. Munves, Ph.D. 125

Introducing New Foods—by Elizabeth D. Munves, Ph.D. 131

A Commonsense Feeding Program—by Walter Sackett, M.D. 135

Toddler Eating Patterns—by Elizabeth D. Munves, Ph.D. 145

Food Allergies—by Elizabeth D. Munves, Ph.D. 151

Allergies (Other Than Foods)—by Elliot Ellis, M.D. 157

SECTION V—Personality and Emotional Development 161

Sibling Rivalry—by Alfred J. Vignec, M.D. 162

Your Baby's Behavior—by Walter J. Coville, Ph.D. 168

Habits—Good and Bad—by Alfred J. Vignec, M.D. 172

Discipline and Punishment—by Alfred J. Vignec, M.D. 180

Your Baby's Personality—by Walter J. Coville, Ph.D. 184

The Aggressive Child—by Alfred J. Vignec, M.D. 189

The Timid Child—by Alfred J. Vignec, M.D. 195

Stuttering—by Jacques P. Penn, Ph.D. 200

Fears in Childhood—by Alfred J. Vignec, M.D. 204

TABLE OF CONTENTS

SECTION VI—Special Health Review 209

Health Record 210

Health Tips—*by R. Cannon Eley, M.D.* 212

Index 230

CONTRIBUTING DOCTORS

ALAN F. GUTTMACHER, M.D.
Obstetrician and Gynecologist
President Planned Parenthood Federation of America, Inc.
Professor Emeritus of Obstetrics—Mt. Sinai School of Medicine, N.Y.C.
Special Lecturer—The College of Physicians & Surgeons, Columbia Presbyterian Medical Center; Albert Einstein College of Medicine and the Harvard University School of Public Health.

HERBERT M. PORTER, M.D., F.A.A.P.
Associate Pediatrician—Lenox Hill Hospital, N.Y.C.

DOROTHY V. WHIPPLE, M.D.
Attending Pediatrician—Children's Hospital, Washington, D.C.
Associate Professor of Clinical Pediatrics, Georgetown University

R. CANNON ELEY, M.D.
Director, Pediatrics Department—Brown University, Providence, R.I.
Chief of Pediatrics—Roger Williams General Hospital, Providence, R.I.

ELIZABETH D. MUNVES, Ph.D.
Professor of Dietetic Medicine,
New Jersey College of Medicine & Dentistry, Newark, N.J.

MELVIN SCHRIER, O.D., F.A.A.O.
Director of the Center for Perceptual Development, N.Y.C.

WALTER J. COVILLE, Ph.D.
Chief, Clinical Psychology Services,
St. Vincent's Hospital, N.Y.C.

CONTRIBUTING DOCTORS

FRANK HOWARD RICHARDSON, M.D., F.A.A.P.
Formerly Regional Consultant to New York Department of Health

MORTON H. WALKER, D.S.C.
Podiatrist and Foot Health Consultant
Author of "Your Guide to Foot Health"

ALFRED J. VIGNEC, M.D.
Former Director of Pediatrics and the
Premature Unit, St. Vincent's Hospital, N.Y.C.
and Medical Director and Pediatrician-in-Chief
of The New York Foundling Hospital

HELEN EVANS REID, M.D.
Research Associate, The Research Institute,
Hospital for Sick Children, Toronto, Canada
and a Registered Specialist in Pediatrics,
Royal College of Physicians and Surgeons of Canada

WALTER W. SACKETT, Jr. M.D.
General Practitioner,
Doctors Hospital, Coral Gables, Fla.

HAROLD SHERMAN, D.D.S.
Assistant Clinical Professor of Restorative Dentistry,
School of Dental and Oral Surgery, Columbia University;
Member of the American Dental Association and the New York Academy of Dentistry

H. LAURENCE DOWD, M.D.
Former Attending Pediatrician at Roosevelt and Doctors
Hospitals, New York City

JACQUES P. PENN, Ph.D.
Adjunct Professor of Speech Pathology and Audiology,
Hunter College, City University of New York, N.Y.C.

SECTION I

Preparing For The Baby

Diet and Weight Control in Pregnancy

by Alan F. Guttmacher, M.D.

THE diet of pregnancy has been the concern of the physician for hundreds of years. The particular foodstuffs which concern him may vary from epoch to epoch yet the focus of concern is always the same—the health of the mother and her unborn baby.

What is the attitude of today's obstetrician toward weight gain and diet during pregnancy?

He insists that the expectant mother's total weight gain during the nine months be restricted to approximately 20 pounds. This limited weight gain not only makes high blood pressure complications less likely but places less strain on the heart.

I am sure, however, that the most appealing argument in favor of restricted weight gain is this—the expectant who gains normally during pregnancy looks infinitely more attractive. She does not have the swollen, gross look which many people associate with the pregnant state.

Ordinarily a few pounds are lost in the early weeks of pregnancy, but they are regained by the end of the third month. From the beginning of the fourth month until a week or two before term, there should be a gradual gain of approximately two pounds every three weeks. The gain is irregular but should never exceed two pounds in one week; if it does the doctor should be notified promptly. A very rapid gain, two pounds or more per week, is ordinarily not due to the accumulation of fat. It is, therefore, not the result of overeating, but is due to the abnormal accumulation of water in all tissues of the body. In such cases, the physician is almost certain to deprive the patient of all free salt (both salt used in the kitchen and salt added at the table) and he is also likely to proscribe all foods rich in salt. Then too, he may give a drug, a diuretic, to aid the elimination of the excess water via the kidneys.

There is an art in weighing one's self correctly. If possible, one should always weigh on the same scale, at the same time wearing the same clothing. The ideal technique is to weigh in the nude before breakfast. A balance scale is preferred to a spring scale.

The idea that the amount of weight gained by the mother affects the birth weight of the baby is probably untrue. Actually the baby is a parasite when it resides within the uterus, and like all parasites, lives and grows at the expense of the host. The ordinary American diet is so well supplied with food essentials that only rarely is an American mother required to sacrifice some of her tissues for her unborn infant.

The diet of pregnancy should be a healthful one—rich in proteins, vitamins and minerals—sparse in fats, starches and carbohydrates. In other words, it is high in body building content and low in calories. You will have to go in training and sit at the anti-obesity table. Unless your husband is long and lean, encourage him to eat the same basic, well-balanced diet you do during pregnancy. He may need less milk, and unless he is trying to slim down, larger servings.

If the prenatal diet is proper, many obstetricians and food experts see no need whatever for dietary supplements in the form of vitamins, iron and other minerals. But on the other hand, if there is a shred of doubt about the adequacy of your diet, dietary supplements are advisable.

The Daily Essentials of a Pregnancy Diet

1. MILK, one quart daily. If the idea of four glasses a day appalls you, cut the bulk in half by dissolving the ingredients of a pint of powdered milk in a pint of whole milk; the result equals a quart. Also you can substitute cheese or ice cream in the proper amount for one or two of the glasses of milk. If you gain too rapidly, your doctor may prefer skimmed milk or fat-free buttermilk over whole milk. If you get leg cramps, it may be advisable to limit the milk to one pint or less and make up the calcium you will lack with some phosphorus-free calcium plus Vitamin D.

2. LEAFY GREEN AND YELLOW VEGETABLES. For a rich source of vitamins A, B and C, and iron, as well as other essential minerals, the green and yellow vegetables are high up on the list of food "musts" for the pregnant woman.

Favorite green vegetables are asparagus, green beans, lima beans, broccoli, Brussels sprouts, green cabbage, chard, endive, kale, leaf lettuce, okra, green peas, spinach, turnip greens, watercress. The best yellow vegetables are carrots, pumpkin, and yellow squash. You should have a minimum of two servings of the above a day—one raw, as a salad.

3. CITRUS FRUITS, TOMATOES and vegetables rich in vitamin C, such as slaw, salad greens, green peppers and turnips, should be served at least twice daily. Canned or frozen juices are satisfactory substitutes for fresh.

4. LEAN MEAT, POULTRY, SEA FOOD AND EGGS. One or two eggs should be included in the daily menu since the yolks are rich sources of iron, vitamins,

and tissue-building proteins. Meat, especially beef, is a perfect food for the pregnant woman and should be eaten at least once a day. Meat bestows fuller nutritive value when not overcooked. Liver and oysters contain a particular blood-building element; one or the other should be on your menu once a week. Poultry, fish and other sea foods are also good sources of animal protein, but not the equal of beef.

5. BREADS AND CEREALS are valuable foods. Whole wheat, dark rye or enriched breads are preferred. Oatmeal, whole corn meal, rye barley, whole wheat-enriched or restored cereals are recommended.

6. POTATOES, OTHER VEGETABLES AND FRUITS also contain valuable minerals and vitamins. Because of greater carbohydrate content, they have higher caloric value than the fruits and vegetables to which reference has previously been made. This makes them more fattening, but since they add variety to the diet and since their bulk also appeases the appetite, they should be eaten (but in moderation).

7. BUTTER OR FORTIFIED MARGARINE. Butter is the best source of vitamin A, but since this vitamin is amply supplied in several of the foods already mentioned, butter is not essential to a well rounded pregnancy diet. If your weight gain is normal, two pats of butter or fortified margarine should be consumed a day.

8. SALT in moderation is permissible in the first half of pregnancy, but should be used sparingly in the second half; salt substitutes can be supplied by your physician. Other condiments can be used as appetite dictates.

9. FLUIDS are essential to health during pregnancy, just as essential as solid foods. The minimum fluid necessary is 2 quarts or 8 glasses a day. Anything which can be poured from glass to glass is counted as fluid; equal credit is given for soup, coffee, fruit juice and milk as for water.

The layman has the idea that in the presence of excessive, rapid weight gain and swollen, water-logged tissues, fluids should be severely restricted. This is not true. As stated earlier, under these conditions, all free salt and salt-containing foods are scrupulously eliminated.

10. MEALS. Frequently three ordinary-sized meals leave the pregnant woman with a full and bloated feeling. If so, she is much better off with six small meals.

A good plan throughout pregnancy is to eat three moderate or slightly skimpy meals, and to raid the ice box in midmorning, midafternoon and just before bedtime. This should be a lady-like raid—the booty being a glass of milk, an apple and a piece of bread and butter, or some crackers and jelly.

These generalizations concerning weight gain and diet during pregnancy may be modified by your own doctor. The statements and rules laid down here are applicable to Mrs. Everywoman. However, to your physician, you are not Mrs. Everywoman—you are you. If he finds you underweight, he may wish you to gain 30 pounds; if overweight, only 5 pounds. Follow his advice. Remember, a competent, interested physician is a trusted guide through the course of your pregnancy.

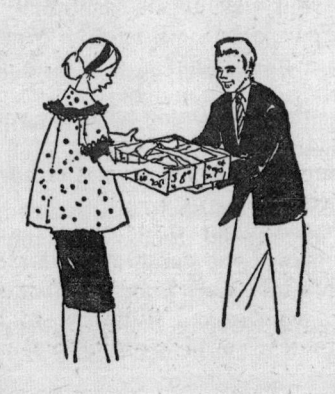

Nutrition and Childbirth

by Elizabeth D. Munves, Ph.D.

ALL mothers wish for a healthy, happy baby. And, during her pregnancy, each mother does her best to create a baby that will be born in the best possible state of health. Yet stories telling of unhappy pregnancies as a result of certain circumstances and events (wholly governed by the choice of the mother) often cause undue anxiety. Each mother may ask herself, "Will this happen to me?"

We are told that losses in the human newborn period are now the third leading medical cause of death in the United States. This data does not include stillbirth, miscarriage, and surviving damaged children. Hepner points out that there is no doubt about the role of nutrition in this problem, but that solid evidence to support this belief has been difficult to marshal.

The infant mortality rate in other parts of the world is considerably higher. Extensive investigations are concerned with identifying the many factors thought responsible. Others are directed toward either reducing or eliminating them.

Many misconceptions are circulated relating nutrition and pregnancy. Such conditions are cleft palate in the baby or other birth defects and malformations, sterility, difficult pregnancies and stillbirths, to name a few, are attributed to deficient diets during pregnancy.

What do we know about the relationship of diet to the outcome of pregnancy? Most individuals are convinced that a "good diet" is important for both the fetus and the mother, but they often wonder how "bad" a poor diet is for all concerned. As might be expected, this is very difficult to determine. Many people ask that such evidence be so-called "black and white", or extreme cases of cause and effect.

Nutrition is only one factor in the development of the baby; there are other equally important ones, such as heredity and other environmental influences. Hepner pointed out that "the interdependence of the many agents known to affect the embryo and fetus is more apparent as investigation continues." An examination of the evidence that does exist will emphasize the difficulty of establishing the exact relationship of nutrition.

Chief among the areas that have been studied are those that are concerned with the process of reproduction, the course of pregnancy, the nutritional status of the mother, the condition of the baby upon birth, and animal experimentation that shows what can take place in other species. Even with this wealth of data, it is difficult to say "this occurred because of this kind of diet or this specific deficiency."

The poor diet patterns found among many teen-age girls has caused considerable concern among many investigators. They feel that the young girls are not storing adequate amounts of nutrients to enter pregnancy in the best possible condition. Their emphasis on the importance of nutritional status prior to conception is supported by studies during World War II on wartime starvation in Holland and Leningrad.

In Holland, the hunger period was one of acute undernutrition that followed four years of regulated but reasonably adequate nutrition. Yet the babies conceived before and born during this period were shorter and weighed less than those born before this period. But the incidence of stillbirth, prematurity and congenital malformation was not increased significantly. The mother's own body stores were able to provide sufficient nutrients to bring the baby to term as she was able to eat fairly well during the pre-starvation period.

This was not true during the siege of Leningrad. Even before the siege, the women were not able to obtain an adequate diet. They were subjected to a state that produced chronic malnutrition of some degree for a long period followed by the acute undernutrition and malnutrition of the siege period. The data about births during this time is significant. The birth rate fell strikingly, and the stillbirth rate doubled. The incidence of prematurity increased to 41%. Death among the full term and the premature babies was considerably higher than normal. Investigators concluded that the nutritional status of the mothers prior to and during pregnancy greatly influenced the health and even the survival of the babies.

Here in the United States extensive studies at Harvard School of Public Health showed that undesirable conditions were found in babies born to those mothers that had poor or very poor prenatal diets. Studies in Great Britain, Scotland and elsewhere in the United States support the importance of the pre-conception diet to successful pregnancy.

Anemia in infancy has been studied in relation to the diet of the mother during pregnancy. A variety of results have been reported, as would be expected. Woodruff stated that full-term infants born of non-anemic mothers normally receive supplies of iron during intrauterine life adequate to meet their requirements for at least three to four months, while infants born to anemic mothers had normal amounts of iron at birth (as measured by hemoglobin levels) yet had developed anemia (hypocromic) at one year. Factors, such as poor iron intake during the first year, can contribute to an anemic state as well as a maternal iron deficiency.

Experiments with animals whereby congenital malformations are produced by nutritional deficiencies are often widely misinterpreted. Action such as this tends to create unnecessary fears in the minds of mothers. Warkany, who has conducted many of these investigations, points out that one of their main contributions to knowledge is to show that malformations that had previously been thought caused by heredity alone can be induced by nutritional deficiencies. He also emphasized that such malformations in man are not due to maternal dietary deficiencies.

Another animal experiment is frequently misrepresented. Because vitamin E is required for normal reproduction in the rat, many erroneously believed that taking vitamin E can relieve sterility in the human. No data is available to support this belief.

Thus, while the negative aspects of poor nutrition are difficult to pinpoint, the positive results can be stated with greater certainty. We can say that with better nutrition more healthy full-term babies will be born. But, because many other factors may be associated with the mother's poor nutritional status (and probably that of the father as well), we cannot conclude that certain specific results are due to poor diets.

Minor Complaints of Pregnancy

by Alan F. Guttmacher, M.D.

A pregnant woman is more prone to physical discomforts than is a nonpregnant woman. Some of these are occasioned by pregnancy; others are exaggerated by it.

Nausea and Vomiting

Since nausea and vomiting are usually mild, confined to the first few waking hours, and self-limited to five or six weeks, they rarely require specific medication. Nevertheless there are a few hints which may prove valuable even for those mildly affected.

Before going to bed place a couple of dry, crisp crackers in a tin box on the bedside table. Upon awakening, eat the crackers without raising your head from the pillow and continue lying on your back for twenty minutes, then get up.

If washing your teeth on arising induces or exaggerates the queasiness, postpone that ritual until later in the day when you feel gastrically stable; in the interim simply rinse your mouth.

If the nausea persists after the dry-cracker routine, eat the following:

1. A light breakfast—for example, oatmeal (or, if preferred, a poached, shirred, or boiled egg); unbuttered toast with marmalade, jelly, or honey; and a cup of coffee or tea.

2. At midmorning, crackers, cake, or toast with a glass of milk or a cup of cocoa.

3. Luncheon, some broth or soup with crackers or toast; rice or a baked potato sprinkled with salt (a baked potato is the nauseated girl's best friend); a salad without oily dressing; and a roll or slice of toast.

4. Midafternoon, crackers, zwieback, or toast with a glass of fruit juice.

5. Dinner, lean meat or seafood; a green vegetable; baked, mashed, or boiled potato; salad; a dessert of ice cream, sherbet, or any other sweet which you feel confident you can keep down; plus bread, toast, or crackers according to taste.

6. Before bed, crackers, cake, or toast with a glass of milk, a cup of cocoa, or a malted milkshake.

Additional fluids should be taken throughout the twenty-four hours. Over a short period fluids are more important to health than solids. Very often iced liquids are best tolerated. Many women in early pregnancy find plain water nauseating, but if a little lemon or orange juice is added it becomes potable. Almost all patients, no matter how nauseated, can take teaspoons of crushed ice flavored by fruit juice, which is a splendid source of fluids. The same may be said for sherbet or water ice, which makes an excellent midafternoon supplement; ginger ale, Coca-Cola, and Pepsi-Cola are valuable drinks since they are rich in carbohydrates.

There are other aids besides diet. Your physician may prescribe a sedative such as ½ grain phenobarbital three or four times a day, or a 10 milligram tablet of Compazine on awakening, and an additional tablet every 6 to 8 hours. If cooking your husband's breakfast aggravates the condition, temporarily cease being domestic. Going out into the air frequently makes you feel better. Don't feel sorry for yourself, keep occupied, and remember the condition is self-limited in duration and almost always a memory by the twelfth week. Keep going; if you have a job, continue working if possible. Carry some crisp salt crackers, graham crackers, or zwieback to munch if a wave of nausea strikes you while on the bus or at the office. Eat small amounts often to prevent your stomach from becoming empty.

The nausea and vomiting of pregnancy usually does not clear up dramatically. Improvement is gradual with the appearance of good days which soon gain the ascendency over the bad days, and then the bad days become fewer and fewer and finally disappear.

A cardinal rule in the control of nausea and vomiting of pregnancy is to avoid foods that you think you cannot keep down, no matter how nutritious and beneficial they are. Substitute any food you think you can retain, no matter whether it is crabmeat or pig's feet. While you are plagued with nausea and vomiting, all the rules of diet are temporarily suspended; but should be in force as soon as the condition clears up.

If you lose ten pounds or more, or find yourself unable to retain any fluids or solids during a twelve-hour period, notify your doctor immediately.

Heartburn

Heartburn, a fiery burning sensation under the middle of the breast bone, is frequently associated with the belching of small amounts of bitter, sour fluid. It may occur in any individual but is most frequently met in pregnant women. The name given to the disorder is a partial misnomer because the condition has nothing to do with the heart but results from sluggish stomach action which delays its emptying, and is a type of indigestion. The omission of rich, greasy foods from the diet—such as mayonnaise, cream, and fried foods—helps, as do smaller and less hurried meals. Relief from heartburn may be gotten by taking a level teaspoon of milk of magnesia or one milk of magnesia tablet after each meal and again whenever heartburn occurs. If this should cause loose stools, substitute other anti-acids such as Maalox, Tums, Rolaids, Titralac, Amphojel, Dijel, or Gelusil. Several come as tablets only, and others in both tablet and liquid form. Do not take bicarbonate of soda, soda mints, or seltzer-type medications because of their high sodium content, which may be injurious during pregnancy. Chewing gum after meals lessens heartburn for some. If heartburn occurs while lying down, sitting up will help. In severe cases do not after meal and when sleeping, elevate the head of the bed with blocks at least one foot high.

Constipation

Some women become constipated only when pregnant, and others prone to constipation find that pregnancy increases the difficulty. The condition results from physiologic changes occurring normally as the effect of pregnancy: decreased contractions of the intestinal tract, pressure from the enlarged uterus on the bowel, and diminished expulsive ability of the overstretched abdominal muscles. The hazards of constipation are greatly overrated in the public mind, probably in part from the emphasis on intestinal hygiene in pharmaceutical advertising in all popular media of communication. There is no evidence of any harm resulting to the patient who does not have a daily bowel movement, except the harm which her propaganda-fired mind imagines. However, an evacuation every twenty-four or forty-eight hours is preferable.

The following regimen will aid constipation:

1. Take a moderate amount of daily physical exercise.
2. Drink at least eight glasses of liquid daily. Drink a glass or two of cold water on arising, and drink one or more glasses of fruit juice during the day.
3. Eat a coarse cereal such as oatmeal for breakfast, and have whole wheat bread in place of white bread. Also eat freely of salads and leafy vegetables.
4. Take some fruit at night before going to bed. Cer-

tain fruits are especially efficacious, notably prunes, apples, figs, dates, and raisins.

5. Licorice candy has a mild cathartic action; take advantage of this property.

6. Try to develop the habit of a regular, unhurried visit to the bathroom at the same hour each day, preferably after breakfast.

7. Refrain from excessive straining while at stool.

When additional measures are necessary, one or two tablespoons of mineral oil nightly before retiring may be tried. This should not be taken during the day because of its interference with the absorption of vitamins and other nutrients. If necessary, a mild laxative such as milk of magnesia or cascara may be taken together with the mineral oil. A popular combination of mineral oil and milk of magnesia is Haley's M-O. Rectal suppositories may be used with impunity if efficacious. Occasional small warm soapsuds enemas are ordinarily permitted unless there has been some complication such as vaginal bleeding or a previous premature delivery. It is safest to consult your doctor before resorting to an enema.

Varicose Veins

Varicose veins are common during pregnancy because of normal physiologic effects, effects which cannot be controlled. Heredity also plays a role; there is a familial tendency toward the occurrence of bad veins which may be transmitted by either parent.

Varicosities are unlikely to appear in a first pregnancy, but when they occur each succeeding baby makes them worse. Fortunately the enlarged veins regress between pregnancies—with the first few pregnancies after their initial appearance, almost completely, but only partially after the later pregnancies. The vessels first involved are most frequently on the inner aspect of the calf, but the process may begin in the space behind the knee or on the thigh, and may involve one leg or both. In the early stages the veins may appear as a spidery network of superficial blood vessels, but when more advanced they stand out as straight, tortuous or knotted, soft blue cords just beneath the skin.

Varicose veins may cause considerable discomfort, usually a dull ache after being on one's feet for some time. Symptoms seem to bear no consistent relationship to the size or the extent of the varicosities.

To reduce the likelihood of developing varicose veins, do not wear round garters or attempt to hold your stockings up by twisting and knotting them about the knee.

If varicose veins develop during pregnancy, several measures may help:

1. Do not stand if you can sit and, when you sit, sit with your leg elevated so that your heel is above the level of the hips. Do not sit if you can lie and, when you lie, lie with your leg raised on a pillow.

2. Use elastic stockings or an ace bandage; either relieves discomfort and probably minimizes the tendency of the varicosities to worsen. Both must be applied before arising, while you are still in bed and the veins are empty. Elastic stockings may be purchased singly or in pairs and should be fitted to both the foot size and leg circumference. They may also be obtained in various lengths, some reaching to just below the knee, others to the groin. It is important that the length be sufficient to cover the uppermost varicosity. The stocking must be held up by a garter belt or girdle. The most satisfactory bandages are made of elastic webbing and are three inches wide and three yards long. In applying the bandage, one or two turns should be made around the foot to anchor it, and then it is wound in a tight spiral around the ankle and up the leg to a point slightly above the highest varicosity. The upper end is fastened by a safety pin or clip. Whether the stocking or bandage is used, it is worn all day and removed at bedtime. Both are washable.

Leg Cramps

Spasm of the calf muscles and muscles of the foot is a common and painful nuisance during pregnancy. The condition is likely to begin about mid-pregnancy, but is usually less frequent the last month. It comes unannounced; most often the patient is aroused from her sleep to find the calf muscles of one leg knotted into a painful, firm ball. The best treatment is local massage, a kneading of the muscle until it relaxes. The area may remain tender for several hours thereafter. Such muscle spasm is not damaging, nor does it denote any abnormality of health. Prevention consists of avoidance of sudden contractions of the leg muscles, not very easy to do, especially if one is asleep. Some physicians recommend adding Vitamin D to the diet and calcium without phosphorus. Before trying either, obtain your doctor's permission.

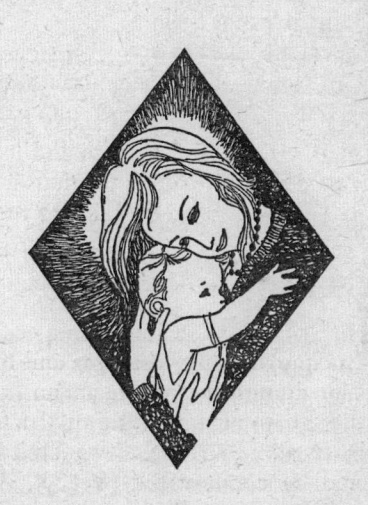

Dental Care For The Expectant Mother

by Harold Sherman, D.D.S.

OVER the centuries, the expectant mother has been the subject of a myriad of superstitions. These "old wives' tales" related to social, medical and dental problems. The dental superstitions have been interesting in that they consist of approximately one per cent fact and about ninety-nine per cent fiction.

Every expectant mother has heard the phrase, "a tooth for every child." The plain implication is that a woman must expect to lose one or more of her teeth every time she bears a child. Many mothers lend credence to this adage by associating the loss of their own teeth with Tim's or Lucy's birth.

Actually, there is a certain element of truth in this superstition, since many mothers have lost teeth during or shortly after pregnancy. But these losses could have been avoided.

We know, for example, that there are hormonal changes during pregnancy, just as there are hormonal changes during puberty and during menstruation. We know also, that these changes do affect the gingival or "gum" tissues of the expectant mother. It has been estimated by dental researchers that a mild form of inflammation of the gums during pregnancy occurs in about fifty per cent of cases. Dentists call this particular type of gum condition "pregnancy gingivitis." In simpler terms, this means that the gums become soft, spongy or puffy and tend to bleed easily. Occasionally the gums between the teeth may swell so extensively as to produce so called "pregnancy tumors."

The important fact to remember is that pregnancy gingivitis is easily treatable by the dentist only with cooperative home care on the part of the patient. It would be wise then for the expectant mother to visit her dentist directly after her first visit to the obstetrician and to inform the dentist of her condition. This first step is very important since simple preventive measures may be taken at this point.

The dentist will very likely remove all foreign matter, such as tartar or impacted food debris from the patient's teeth and gums. This will immediately eliminate focal points of irritation which, later, would aggravate any weakened condition of the gums. He may decide to close open contact spaces between the teeth, since such spaces may cause chronic food impactions and the consequent disturbance of the gums. The dentist may then advise his patient on the proper home care of her teeth and gums. This care may vary from correct tooth-brushing to a variety of techniques of stimulating her gums—if the latter is required. Finally, the dentist may call to the attention of the expectant mother the important relationship of diet and dental health. A well-balanced diet yielding all of the essential nutrient factors in adequate amounts is essential for the development and maintenance of gum tissues, just as it is essential for the health of other body tissues.

If the expectant mother visits her dentist early enough to permit preventive care, the fairly common problem of "pregnancy gingivitis" need not lead to the loss of teeth. In fact, such prophylactic measures may possibly prevent the development of "pregnancy gingivitis," or at least reduce it to a very innocuous condition.

Another more direct cause of loss of teeth among expectant mothers is dental decay. There are two areas of misinformation on this subject. One is that pregnancy causes dental decay. The other is that it is dangerous to have dental work performed during pregnancy.

The fallacy of the first belief has been demonstrated by many dental researchers, including the late Dr. Daniel Ziskin, of the School of Dental and Oral Surgery, Columbia University. In 1937, Dr. Ziskin and Dr. Hotelling reported (on a study that was based on a group of 324 pregnant women, with pregnancies ranging from one to eight months) that "pregnancy, per se, is not a cause of dental caries (decay)."

However, the expectant mother may develop cavities as a result of poor oral hygiene—coincidentally with the period of pregnancy, or she may have a backlog of untreated dental decay of pre-pregnancy vintage. Regardless of the source of the cavities, she may then be concerned with the safety of dental procedures required to treat the decayed teeth. Here, of course, we have a major source of unnecessary loss of teeth. The misinformed expectant mother shuns dental treatment because of unwarranted fears, and thereby may shortly lose one or more teeth that could have been saved in routine fashion. Dentists have found that dental treatments of all kinds can be performed in most cases, without danger to the pregnancy.

Some mothers are not so much concerned with the "drilling" or excavating of cavities as they are with the possible ill effects of the local anesthetic (novocaine injection) or general anesthetic ("gas") that is often employed. A reassuring statement on this matter may be found in the report of Dr. K. L. Schupp, in the California State Dental Journal of September, 1941: "In the past six years at the prenatal clinic at San Francisco Hospital, our dentists have made 5,371 examinations and made 3,300 extractions. In none of these cases, all of which had an anesthetic, local or general, was there any accident, miscarriage, or any other untoward accident. This eliminates any cause for fear that such procedures have a bad effect upon the course of pregnancy."

It should be clear from the foregoing discussion that pregnancy may cause a temporary mild gingivitis which is easily treatable, that pregnancy does not cause dental decay, and that all kinds of dental treatment of the prenatal patient are not only safe, but necessary and important.

We may therefore conclude that the expectant mother should consult her family dentist soon after her first visit to the obstetrician. Thus the dentist will have adequate time to restore decayed teeth, to treat, preventively, susceptible gums, institute proper home care and to review the importance of a well-balanced diet to good dental health.

The wise expectant mother will take such measures and thereby obviate the possibility of losing "a tooth for every child."

For A Healthy Pregnancy

by **Alan F. Guttmacher, M.D.**

I wish to make the clear-cut, unqualified statement that the directions included here are intended in no way to displace or alter those of the reader's physician. There are great differences of informed opinion on the lesser details of the conduct of normal pregnancy. Further, every obstetrician's treatment will vary in detail to suit variations in individual patients. No matter how carefully a pregnant woman may study this or any other book, she will not obviate the necessity of paying an early visit to her physician.

It is remarkable how life during pregnancy has been simplified in recent years. With the observation of large numbers of healthy women—previous to the eighteenth century midwives cared for all normal cases, and doctors had the opportunity to see only ill pregnant women—the medical attitude toward pregnancy has changed. Since in the pre-modern era pregnancy was treated as an illness (from its very inception) it was deemed imperative to employ the most complicated measures to prevent dangerous complications. We now realize that pregnancy is a normal, simple physiologic state, and ordinarily all that need be done is to maintain the woman in good physical and psychological condition by the enforcement of an uncomplicated, commonsense regimen. If an abnormality develops, then, of course, the doctor must step in and aid nature to correct it.

Exercise

The previously held conviction that practically anything except lying alone in bed might bring on abortion or premature labor must have been devastating to both mind and conscience. Until very recently, whenever a woman miscarried she searched her life for the cause, and with no difficulty, discovered it either in some minor accident or in the simple exertions of her everyday existence. With advances in knowledge concerning the real causes of abortion, our attitude toward exercises during pregnancy has changed. We realize that the majority of miscarriages are blessed acts on the part of nature to terminate further development of an abnormal ovum.

Most physicians allow their patients any form of exercise throughout pregnancy: swimming, tennis, dancing, golf, hiking, and horseback riding. Other physicians, adopting the more conservative course, allow only milder forms of exercise, especially during the first three months, when miscarriage is most common. I belong to the former group, the any-exercise-within-moderation school.

Travel

There are only two arguments against travel during pregnancy:

1. Abortion or labor can happen at any hour on any day, and it is nearly always impossible to predict the occurrence. If the pregnant woman happens to be traveling at the time of such an emergency, or is residing in a community other than her own, it is both inconvenient and frightening. One way to lessen the difficulty is to ask your doctor to furnish you with the name of an obstetrician colleague living in the area you plan to visit. Put the memorandum in your handbag and expect not to need it—almost certainly you will not.

2. Traveling can be fatiguing and uncomfortable, especially in late pregnancy. This is particularly true of automobile travel. The only antidote is to break up the

trip every one hundred to a hundred and fifty miles, get out of the car, void, and walk about for a few minutes. It is unwise for the pregnant woman to motor more than three hundred miles a day.

Decisions as to mode of travel during pregnancy should be governed mainly by commonsense considerations. For example, if the woman is prone to motion sickness, the train is probably best. Long distances are usually accomplished with the least fatigue and discomfort by air. Many commercial airlines require a physician's letter to allow travel during the last three months. Air travel during the first three months has been subjected to recent discussion on the basis that lessened oxygen at this critical, formative period of the fetus's development might in the rare case be the cause of a fetal abnormality. With the well-pressurized commercial planes of today, I see no reason *not* to fly in early pregnancy.

Automobile Driving

It is not injurious for the pregnant woman to drive herself, and she may continue to do so as long as she can sit comfortably behind the wheel. During the last trimester it is inadvisable that she drive alone at night, or on little frequented roads, because of the potential problems that might arise from a flat tire or other automotive emergencies. Unless a car is equipped with power steering, urban parking may be very exhausting, and this should be taken into account during the late months of pregnancy.

Pregnancy is a poor time to learn to drive, because of the clumsiness sometimes associated with it and the possible slowing of reactions from lessened powers of concentration. Also a serious accident may be compounded by the pregnant state.

Sleep and Rest

In early pregnancy the average woman requires an

unusually large amount of sleep; this need disappears between the twelfth and sixteenth weeks. The last months are marked by sleeplessness, mainly due to difficulty in finding a comfortable position. Frequently, I am asked if it is harmful to sleep on the back or stomach. No possible harm can result from any position, since the fetus is so well protected that pressure does not affect it. Pregnant women are often convinced that the fetus is nocturnal in its habits and with studied malice chooses nighttime to cut capers. The doctor disagrees, for he thinks that the woman simply has a greater opportunity to feel the movements at this time, since nothing diverts her attention. As there is no way to diminish the fetal movements, the only remedy is a hypnotic (prescribed by the doctor) that will make the woman sleep, despite them. The amount of sleep should be governed by habit and desire, the safest rule being to sleep enough to awake well rested. The best health insurance during pregnancy is an hour's bedrest in a darkened room late each afternoon; with the rest before dinner, food tastes better, life appears rosier, and late evening hours are more happily tolerated.

If you are sleeping poorly, discuss it with your doctor. He will go over your bed habits and make some valuable suggestions, or perhaps prescribe a hypnotic.

Smoking. Cigarette smoking is unwise at all times and particularly during pregnancy. Strangely enough, infants of heavy smokers (more than one pack a day) average about 12 ounces less at birth than the babies of nonsmokers. They are carried the same length of time in both groups but are just smaller in size among babies of smokers. This weight deficit does not adversely effect either survival or later development of the baby nor is it associated with an increase in congenital abnormalities. If you must smoke, try to limit your cigarettes to 10 or less a day while you are pregnant. Cigarette smoking speeds up the fetal heart, but this does no harm since the heart rate returns to normal after you have finished your cigarette.

Alcohol. The moderate use of alcohol neither affects the maternal nor fetal health during pregnancy. Alcohol is excreted in the mother's milk providing the baby with a milk punch which in excess may mildly inebriate the infant.

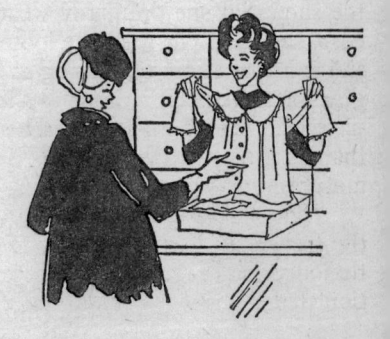

Care of the Feet During Pregnancy

by **Morton H. Walker, D.S.C.**

THE feet and their effect on posture influence the internal organs of a woman. Like other organs, the uterus is subjected to gravitational pull. When this pull is altered by weak, imbalanced feet, excessive stress is placed on the cervical attachments and injury may be caused to the uterus.

Pregnancy itself puts a strain on the uterus. But when this strain is compounded by poor posture and weak feet, then the pregnant woman will suffer.

During pregnancy it is very important to make sure the feet are strong and able to carry the extra burden. Shoes play a role. Any shoe that is extreme is condemned. A pregnant woman should not wear a high heel, pointed toe shoe that she ordinarily wears during her social life. Also, she must not wear the loose, flat, casual shoe which she is in the habit of wearing at home. The proper footgear for a pregnant woman is a leather sole, rubber heel, six eyelet oxford made of leather and having not higher than an inch and a half heel. This kind of shoe is not the most fashionable, but it is the healthiest.

The shoe should be fitted at the end of the day when the feet are at their fullest. It should be fitted just a little longer and a little wider so as to take into consideration that the feet may swell more as pregnancy advances.

You definitely cannot wear the same shoes you usually wear. Pregnancy is a "different" state. The costume you wear is different too, and whereas you wear maternity clothes, you should wear maternity shoes.

You should give attention to any unusual excrescences on the feet at this time. Corns, calluses, warts or ingrown nails should be eliminated as much as possible. It is important to keep the feet pain-free so that unusual gait or stance will be avoided. That way you will not put excessive stress on muscles, ligaments and bones that already are carrying an extra amount of weight. These rules for foot health must be followed:

1. Keep the feet clean by washing or soaking them at least once a day.

2. Powder the feet with a good absorbent commercial brand of foot powder every day, and especially after the foot bath.

3. Cut the toenails straight across and avoid clipping the corners of the nails.

4. Scrape hard skin with a pumice stone or light sandpaper so there is no accumulation to cause pain.

5. Visit your podiatrist at least once a month during the prenatal period to get his advice and to make sure you maintain good foot health.

Elastic stockings are called for when varicose veins show signs of occurring. The little spider web formations that appear as red blotches on the legs are warning signs and should not be ignored. Elastic stockings should come up above the knees. They must be strong and of a narrow mesh. The sheerer quality is all right. The stockings should be washed daily and allowed to dry on a sock or stocking stretcher.

Gentle foot exercise done for five minutes a day will reap its own reward. Pick up marbles with your toes and walk around the room with them. While sitting, rotate the ankles gently in one direction and then in another. Walk on the toes for a minute or two or stand on one

CARE OF THE FEET DURING PREGNANCY

leg and swing the other back and forth a few times. Walking barefoot on soft surfaces such as beach sand or lawns is wonderful exercise for the small foot muscles. This is even good on a deep pile rug, but avoid walking barefoot on flat hard surfaces like asphalt tile, hardwood floors or concrete pavements. When climbing up or down stairs, go slowly, walk steadily and watch where you walk.

Do not walk barefoot in the dark. Injuries to the toes by banging them on pieces of furniture are easy when you can't see where you're going. A fractured toe, although not serious, will only complicate your pregnancy and make you more uncomfortable.

Occasionally use lubricating cream on your feet. Remember the skin on the foot is just like the hands, and it needs attention too. If you will treat your feet as you treat your hands, they will take care of you with no problems.

Foot care is important during pregnancy, perhaps as important as keeping your weight down. If your feet hurt, you won't feel like accomplishing the many little jobs in preparation for the blessed event. You will have to force yourself to accept motherhood and you will not like being forced one bit.

Management of Twin Pregnancy

by Alan F. Guttmacher, M.D.

THERE are several things which make one's doctor suspect the possibility of twins. First, a uterus larger than one would expect in view of the duration of pregnancy. For example, ordinarily the top of the uterus reaches just below the navel at 20 weeks. Suppose the uterus is an inch or two above the navel, then it is probably either twins, one very large baby, excessive fluid in the sac surrounding the child (hydramnios) or the dates are wrong. With twins the uterus, in addition to being high, is often very broad. Second, when on abdominal examination the doctor thinks he palpates (feels) an excessive number of small parts, that is, feet or hands, or two heads or two breeches (buttocks). Third, excessive weight gain. This is most likely due to overeating or to abnormal retention of tissue fluid, (edema). However, in a betting pool, buy a ticket on twins for "show." Fourth, if relatively early in pregnancy, by the thirty-second or thirty-third week, the doctor feels a small head already deep in the pelvis, probably due to the excessive internal uterine pressure which normally occurs with a multiple pregnancy. I recall that I made this point one evening several years ago at a medical lecture. The next morning at 7 a.m. the telephone rang in my hotel room, much to my displeasure, and a cheerful, wide-awake voice said, "Good morning, doctor. I want to congratulate you before you leave. You know last night as you spoke about a small head entering the pelvis early, I remembered a patient whom I had seen yesterday afternoon who had just that. I could hardly wait for the talk to be over. I rushed to the telephone and called her and said, 'Phyllis, come down to the office at once. I think you may have twins.' She came down at 10:30 last night and doctor, she had them. I was able to hear two fetal hearts."

This leads me quite positively to a doctor's positive diagnosis of twins, rather than his suspicion. First, if he can hear over the abdomen (usually by means of his stethescope) two hearts beating at rates ten beats or more apart. This difference prevents him from mistaking a single heart beat audible over two different areas of the abdomen for two hearts. The two heart beats of a pair of twins usually can be heard by about the twenty-second to twenty-sixth week of pregnancy. Second, a well-equipped laboratory can make a fetal electrocardiogram and register two different fetal tracings. This can occasionally be done as early as the twelfth and almost always by the sixteenth or eighteenth week. Third, an abdominal X-ray showing two fetal skeletons is almost always positive by the sixteenth week.

Suppose the diagnosis of twins is made, what is done about it? Each doctor has his own rules and for you, his rules are better than mine. However here are mine: 1) Get more rest than if you were carrying one; or ease your job, if you have one. A nap in midafternoon is good twin assurance.

2) Remove salt from your diet. However, you may use one of several salt substitutes. This is done to diminish the tendency, which twin mothers, have of retaining water in the tissue (edema). It also reduces the likelihood of a high blood pressure complication.

3) Watch your weight. Even with twins do not gain more than 30 pounds; 25 pounds is a better maximum.

4) Take the iron pills which no doubt your physician will prescribe when he knows you have twins, as anemia is more likely to develop in a twin than a single pregnancy.

5) See your doctor frequently. Very probably from the thirtieth week on he will require you to visit him at least once a week. It is likely he will give you an internal examination at each visit to determine whether the mouth of the womb (cervix) is beginning to shorten or to dilate. If this occurs before the thirty-sixth week, no doubt he will confine you to bed at home or in the hospital to reduce the risk of premature labor, a common complication of twin pregnancy.

6) Notify your doctor at once if the waters break, pains begin or you spot or bleed.

An average set of twins arrives three weeks earlier than a single baby; therefore, if your twin labor begins a month or so early, don't be surprised.

Rh (Erythroblastosis)

by R. Cannon Eley, M.D.

"RARELY has it been our good fortune to have a disease recognized, its cause clearly determined, its treatment successfully developed to a great extent, and then its prevention found, all in one generation." This is a quotation from a famous medical publication (Pediateics, January, 1968) from an article by Dr. Louis K. Diamond, internationally recognized authority on blood disorders in infants and children, and one of the pioneers in the study of Rh.

The disease to which Dr. Diamond refers in the quotation is medically known as "erythroblastosis fetalis." It is actually caused by an incompatibiity between the mother's blood and the blood of the unborn infant, which results in a lack of red blood cells in the newborn.

Treating babies with this disease has been a serious medical problem for many years. In 1946 "exchange transfusions" were introduced to save the baby's life. By this procedure some of the baby's blood is withdrawn and replaced by a blood free from substances that will destroy the Rh positive blood cells. When this transfusion treatment was initiated, the mortality rate among newborn babies was reduced, but it was very risky and difficult. A further attempt was made in 1962, when a method of transfusing babies during pregnancy was developed by Dr. A. W. Wiley of New Zealand. This still further reduced the death rate among newborn infants but could only be used in special cases.

What is the Rh factor that causes this death-inducing disease among infants? Perhaps no condition of pregnancy has been so much discussed and so badly misunderstood. These two seemingly innocent letters (Rh) have given rise to much fear and worry among expectant mothers.

The fact remains, however, that Rh has caused the deaths of almost 10,000 infants in the United States every year.

The Rh factor is an inherited substance in the blood. It was so named because it was first discovered in the blood of the Rhesus monkey (in which the Rh factor is always present.) Eighty-five per cent of the American and European white people have this factor in their blood; these people are called Rh positive. The other fifteen per cent (who do not have it) are called Rh negative. The Rh factor can be transmitted from parents to children in a variety of ways—but the possession of, or lack of, Rh in the blood has no effect whatever on health, vigor or longevity.

Problems can arise when an Rh positive husband is married to an Rh negative wife. If a baby inherits his father's Rh positive factor and his mother is Rh negative, there is a chance that blood disease may develop in the infant. Trouble can arise when the unborn baby's Rh positive blood cells sensitize the blood of the Rh negative mother through the placenta. If the baby's Rh blood enters the mother's bloodstream, she fights it by manufacturing an antibody. It is when the mother's antibodies bypass the placenta and enter the bloodstream of a subsequent baby that the baby's red blood cells are destroyed, and the resulting Rh disease may cause anemia, jaundice, brain damage, or even death.

First babies run little risk of Rh; it is in subsequent births that the antibodies (developed by the mother

RH (ERYTHROBLASTOSIS)

after her first child was delivered) can do the greatest harm.

Among the new and miraculous break-throughs in medicine is the development of an anti-Rh gamma globulin obtained from the blood plasma of Rh-negative volunteers who have been sensitized by pregnancy, and thereby carry the antibody against Rh positive blood cells. To prevent sensitization, this vaccine-like drug is given to an Rh negative mother within 72 hours following the birth, or miscarriage, of her first Rh positive child. Furthermore, it must be repeated after each subsequent birth of a baby with the Rh positive factor. Once the mother has become sensitized, and has developed antibodies that will destroy the red blood cells of the baby, this vaccine is of no value. So there may still remain a need for transfusions during pregnancy.

Your obstetrician will discuss this new globulin with you; there are certain tests which he will make to determine whether your blood characteristics and those of your baby meet the requirements for these injections.

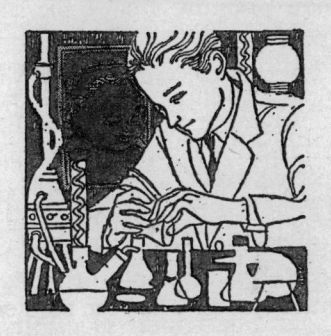

The Father's Role

by Alan F. Guttmacher, M.D.

TODAY, among us, a husband's chief assignment during pregnancy and birth is to provide emotional support for his wife. This behind-the-scenes function gives him an important career to work at—one that is second only to his chosen vocation.

Along with it, however, goes fourth billing in the cast—mother, baby, obstetrician and then father-to-be. Such secondary status for the father is not universal.

Among some primitive groups, the laboring, groaning father is given medical assistance while the stoical childbearing mother is ignored. This curious custom is termed "couvade" (from the French word "couver" meaning to hatch)—or man-childbed. In British Guiana, the woman works until she goes into labor, but some days before the expected event the father takes to his hammock. He is prohibited certain foods for fear they may cause the child to be lean, and other foods lest they cause its teeth to be crooked. When labor begins, the wife goes silently into the woods while the man groans in his hammock of pain. She returns soon after the child is born and during the lying-in period, the next ten days, she must take care of the father, herself and the baby.

Couvade, or traces of couvade, have been found on every continent. There are several explanations, but no one knows the true reason. One possibility is that couvade is intended to deceive evil spirits, witches and demons. Since at birth, both the mother and child are in peril, the father, by making the groans of travail and exhibiting other symptoms of labor, creates the illusion that he is bringing forth the child. The evil influences then concentrate upon him, allowing the woman to bear her child in safety. Another explanation may be the father's desire in a matriarchal society to emphasize the blood bond between himself and his offspring.

The only instance of couvade I have encountered is nausea and vomiting during early pregnancy by a highly sympathetic husband. Other physicians have observed the same thing. Pregnancy nausea and vomiting by the father carries the idea of emotional support a little too far. It is important to let the wife feel that her husband cares, but not to this extent.

What can a father-to-be do to be a partner in this most important event? He can share his wife's enthusiasm; he must realize that every mother-to-be thinks that no one will ever produce such an important child. Then too, he can read and study about pregnancy and birth with his wife. As the author of a popular book, I can attest that many husbands become amateur obstetricians. Not infrequently a husband says to me, "Dr. Guttmacher, this and this happened exactly as you said in your book."

At many hospitals, classes for expectant parents are addressed to the couple. Day-classes are attended by the mother alone, and a few evening meetings are attended by the mother-and-father-to-be together. There are also night groups in which couples attend *all* sessions together. The husbands ask searching questions proving they think seriously about impending fatherhood.

During pregnancy a father-to-be can give his wife emotional support by making fewer demands, such as preparing his breakfast when she feels ill or weary. Then too, he can build her morale by a well-timed compliment on the new becoming pregnancy look. He should encourage joint pleasant social activities and discourage their becoming recluses. If the doctor imposes some dietary restrictions such as no potatoes or no sweet desserts, it is far easier if the husband also goes on the diet. This removes temptation which may defeat his wife's will-power.

There is still division of medical opinion about the safety of sexual intercourse during pregnancy. A small segment of physicians forbid it throughout the nine months—an unnecessary and impractical recommendation, in my view. Others urge that it be omitted during the days of the month when the first few menstrual periods would be due. In the absence of vaginal bleeding or a history of repeated miscarriages, sexual intercourse is permissible, desirable, and safe at any time during pregnancy until four weeks before the expected delivery date—unless, of course, there has been premature rupture of the membranes.

If there is vaginal discomfort, preliminary lubrication with vaseline or cold cream may be helpful. When there is any staining or bleeding after sexual intercourse, sex relations should be abandoned completely until the doctor is consulted. If the wife finds the usual position during intercourse uncomfortable, some variation in positioning may be indicated.

Most wives want their husband with them or near them during labor. We encourage a husband to sit with his wife in the hospital during the first part of labor. I have witnessed all kinds of joint activities such as crossword puzzles, recording the length of contractions and the interval between them, or reading aloud to each other.

In some hospitals, particularly those which welcome Natural Childbirth, the husband accompanies his wife into the delivery room. After he is masked, capped and gowned, he stands by his wife at the head of the delivery table and usually holds her hand or strokes her forehead. Above all, he keeps out of the way. If the wife is given general anesthesia, the husband leaves before she falls into unconscious sleep.

Following delivery, the husband is busy spreading the good tidings. He is usually provided with a pre-delivery list of relatives and special friends to telephone and telegraph—which is a wonderful outlet for his happy, exuberant spirits.

Sometimes a new mother has "the blues" after her delivery or during the first weeks at home with her new baby. Periods of depression and crying without cause are common at these times. If the father is aware of this, he can be a great comfort to his wife. For one thing, he can be patient and understanding when she seems weepy and on edge. For another, he can be a strong, steadying influence, a pillar of strength for her to lean on until she gets her emotions on an even keel.

Of course when the baby comes home from the hospital, there is plenty the father can do. A bottle-fed baby loves to take the 2 a.m. bottle from Daddy and the newborn admires the authoritative way he pins diapers. Dad also excels at bathing the baby. Having a baby is a partnership job. Fathers-to-be, pay heed!

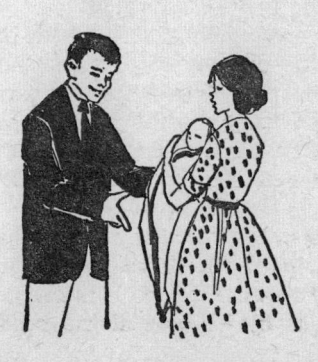

Advice to New Mothers

by Alan F. Guttmacher, M.D.

THE following are my own rules for the new mother during the first few weeks after leaving the hospital. However, I again issue the sincere warning that if the rules which follow differ from your own doctor's, utterly disregard mine and follow his scrupulously.

On the day before the new mother leaves the hospital I give her the following farewell speech. It is meant only for the normal case who has had an uncomplicated vaginal delivery and in whom convalescence has been uninterrupted. The patient delivered by Caesarean section, or who had some complication, receives different instructions.

This is my advice to her:

"Your case was delightfully normal. When you go home tomorrow, walk up the steps. More people are killed by being carried up than walking up.

"Stay on the same floor for three or four days after getting home from the hospital, if convenient. If not, you may go downstairs once a day, perhaps for dinner; if you do, you might as well stay downstairs for the evening. Rest for most of the afternoon, if possible sleeping for two hours.

"When you have been home for three or four days, reduce the afternoon rest to two hours. On the same day you do this, you may walk downstairs and if the weather is nice, go outdoors for a five minute stroll. The next day you may go out a little longer; each day increase your activities. When you have been home ten days, you may do nearly what you please—go downtown to a movie, go out to dinner, do light housework, etcetera. Don't take on heavy household duties until the baby is three or four weeks old.

"You may ride in a car when the baby is two weeks old and drive it yourself when the baby is four weeks old.

"You may eat, drink and smoke what you want. If you are breast feeding, you must drink a quart of milk each day and go lightly on cigarettes and drinking, for both nicotine and alcohol are excreted in the milk—perhaps nature's attempt to build up tolerance early in life.

"You may take a full bath as soon as you get home, and bathe at least once a day. If stitches or hemorrhoids pain you, the more often you bathe the better. You may douche after the baby is three weeks old if you wish to, but it is rarely necessary. If you decide to douche, use a can or bag and lie with your hips elevated in the bath tub. I would not douche more often than every other day.

"Wear any clothing which is comfortable. Do not wear a girdle constantly, since it acts like a splint to the abdominal muscles and retards them from getting their tone back.

"Make an engagement to see me in my office when the baby is five or six weeks old, and don't have intercourse until I check you. Come alone—leave the baby at home."

SECTION II

Caring For The Newborn

The New Arrival

by Alfred J. Vignec, M.D.

THE average young mother looks forward eagerly during the long and at times tedious months of pregnancy to the moment when her own new baby will be placed in her arms. This prenatal period is extremely important from a psychological point of view. It is during this time that the mother should make several vital decisions. Should she breast feed the baby or place him on a prepared product or standard formula? Will she plan to keep him on a relatively fixed schedule or allow him more latitude in his feeding habits? Will she use rooming-in facilities, if her hospital has them available? Many of these questions should be answered before the baby comes and for this reason, it would be wise for more prospective mothers, particularly first-time mothers, to visit their pediatricians as well as their obstetricians before delivery. (This, however, is not a general practice, and most mothers meet their pediatricians for the first time at the hospital after the baby has arrived.)

Once the baby is born, almost miraculously the long months of waiting and indeed even the hours of labor are erased from the mother's mind. She is almost euphoric, talking about her baby and displaying him eagerly to her family and friends. It seems that all should be happiness for her now, with no cloud to mar the future. Why then the "baby blues?" In large part, of course, the reason for this at times distressing let-down is physiological. The body has been taxed by the stresses of pregnancy and delivery, there have been hormonal changes, etc. But partly, too, the same small stranger who is so warmly welcomed is himself the cause of this distress.

Small things begin to appear to disturb the mother. When she really inspects her baby she notices that his head is not quite symmetrical, that his skin and even the whites of his eyes may be tinged with yellow. The head, of course, has been molded during his passage through the birth canal and will quite normally readjust itself in time; the slightly yellow color is physiological jaundice and will disappear in a few days. Doctors and nurses at the hospital clarify these matters, and the mother is reassured until one day he appears with his mouth and lips purple! Actually this is only gentian violet which is applied routinely in many hospitals as a precautionary measure against thrush (fairly often found in newborn babies and very easily controlled). But in her somewhat precarious emotional condition, the mother may be upset by it.

The baby seems so fragile. He cries readily and without warning and cannot understand her words of comfort. The small mouth clamps tightly against the nipple at times in refusal. If feeding is forced, he regurgitates. Occasionally he will not burp and squirms in pain or frowns in his sleep, and she feels powerless to deal with the discomfort of such a small being.

While the mother is still in the hospital, there is always someone to turn to. But it must be borne in mind that the modern hospital stay is relatively short and the task of carrying the baby through his first few weeks of adjustment to life falls almost entirely on the mother. While it is true that she receives advice from her pediatrician, the details are often lost in the excitement of departure for home, and she finds herself in some confusion. She may even surrender to tears, much to the consternation of her family. The tears are not significant, nor should they be alarming. The slight physiological depression will pass. However, the more information the mother can collect, the better she will be equipped to cope with the problems of the new baby.

Does the baby see, hear, taste, feel pain? Yes, he hears. Loud noises may alarm him. Some infants quiet down when music is played, also in response to the crooning voice of the mother. To all appearances, he has some sense of taste, as bitter or excessively salty or obnoxious substances cause grimacing. However, his taste is not selective during this first phase. He also sees, vaguely—light and dark, shapes, and by one month of age, some movement. His sense of pain is less acute the younger he is. Early circumcision, for example, can be done without anesthesia with little discomfort. However, the infant dislikes restraints, and can be made to cry if his head or limbs are held, even gently.

Will his hair fall out? It may. In fact, an infant born with a considerable amount of hair may become completely bald. This is not unnatural. Nor are crosseyes. During the period when the infant is learning to focus, particularly during the first two months, the eye muscles are weak and complete crossing of the eyes, or strabismus, is common. The infant may also sneeze frequently and have hiccups. This, too, is a part of adaptation to his new environment.

What about his cord? Shortly after his arrival home (up to ten days or two weeks of age, usually) the cord will dry up and drop off. Once it is off and dry, the infant may be bathed and taken out, in weather above freezing (32 deg. Fahrenheit). He should be dressed adequately but not too warmly, as heat rash brought on by overzealous mothers is not uncommon even in mid-winter. Should the cord scar remain moist, the pediatrician may be consulted and will probaby apply an astringent to promote drying.

May he lie on his stomach? Yes, if pillows and soft bedding are not placed in such a way that the infant can smother or strangle. He is not strong enough at first to move his own head to a position of safety.

What about his feeding? If the mother is breast feeding her physician will instruct her. If the infant is on formula, nipple hole sizes are of primary importance to the infant's comfort and well-being. The nipple hole may be enlarged with a hot sewing needle. It should be large enough to permit the warm milk to drip as fast as possible without forming a stream. If smaller, the infant frustrates himself—if larger, he may develop colic. Must he finish every bottle? Not necessarily. Often an infant leaves an ounce or two and makes it up at the next feeding. A baby who is forced is often also a baby who regurgitates. Must he burp after every two ounces? He should, but not necessarily "must." At times he may refuse. Again, excessive pounding may cause regurgitation. Vitamins should be administered conscientiously in the prescribed quantities. Their importance does not diminish until at least adolescence and it is wise to continue them even beyond this age. They are useful supplements even to an adult diet.

One more item worthy of mention in connection with feeding—the mother should not discourage easily if her baby "does not care for" solids. Fruits often go well, as they are sweet and palatable, but most infants take quite a while to accustom themselves to the flavor and texture of strained vegetables and meats. The baby may use various methods of acquainting the mother with the fact that he prefers fruit to anything else—he may "smack" his lips over fruit and "complain" about other things, or simply spit out the vegetables and meat, or close his mouth. However, gentle persistence in offering these foods without forcing usually succeeds, and after several months the infant accepts one food as readily as another. If the mother gives up too soon she lays the foundation for future feeding problems. It is always wise to remember that the infant begins to form his patterns of behavior at birth, if not before. Cuddle him and comfort him, give him as much affection as possible so that he will feel secure and loved—but if he is picked up whenever he cries, he will very soon cry to be picked up.

It is impossible, of course, to cover all situations which the mother may encounter with her new infant in so short an article, but several general rules may prove helpful:

1. If in serious doubt about anything concerning the infant's physical status or behavior, the mother should consult her pediatrician.

2. If the matter does not seem important enough to seek outside advice the mother should use her own judgment. With a second child, she has already acquired so much confidence that she automatically thinks for herself, and is usually right. For example, if the weather is so cold that she cannot walk the baby without discomfort, it is also too cold for the baby to be out. If her hands are cold, he needs mittens. If she goes hatless, in a sweater, he does not need a heavy jacket and a wool cap. In other matters the same type of reasoning is helpful.

3. The baby is not as fragile as he looks. His head must be carefully supported at all times until his neck muscles are strong enough for him to take over. But he is not "breakable" and with reasonable care, can very safely be handled.

Before long the mother's physical condition is improved, she gains in confidence and strength, and the baby no longer seems a stranger. It is truly amazing how quickly he becomes a small person with likes and dislikes, modes of expression and faith in the mother who is his caretaker.

Diaper Rash

by R. Cannon Eley, M.D.

DIAPER rash, otherwise known as "ammoniacal diaper rash" gets its name from the fact that the eruption or rash appears over that area of the body covered by the diaper, i.e., the lower abdomen, genitalia, and inner areas of the thighs and buttocks. It is most commonly found among infants over two months old who are exposed to wet diapers for a prolonged period of time.

As the name implies, "ammoniacal diaper rash" is caused by ammonia in the urine which irritates the skin. It is not caused as some people think by something in the baby's diet. The ammonia is produced by the presence of certain bacteria which originate in the intestines, and which bring about chemical changes in the urine on baby's skin.

It naturally follows that the longer a wet diaper remains on the baby, and the more saturated it becomes from repeated voiding, the more severe the rash. Body heat, perspiration, clothing and waterproof pants can all help to aggravate the condition, producing raw, red, "scalded," often blistered and painful skin.

Actually diaper rash itself is not the greatest problem; a definite danger lies in the possibility of secondary infection of the skin by bacteria, or by a fungus such as monilia (thrush) or yeast. In circumcised male infants, repeated diaper rashes (and especially severe ones) may so irritate the opening of the penis through which the urine is voided that ulcerations are produced. When healed, they may cause such a narrowing of this opening that voiding becomes difficult. Such a condition presents a real problem. It might be well if doctors considered this hazard before advocating circumcision of all newborn male infants before they leave the hospital. Circumcision can be performed after the diapering period just as well as during it.

The best treatment for diaper rash is its prevention —and this can be accomplished by several means. As ordinary home washing does not remove the ammonia from the fibers of the fabric, the diapers should be boiled after thorough washing with soap and water—and finally rinsed in water to which has been added an antiseptic that will inhibit or prevent the growth of the bacteria that produces ammonia. Diapers should be wrung out lightly, thus allowing some of the antiseptic to remain in the material, and allowed to dry, in the sun, if possible. Many antiseptic products are poisons and should be kept out of reach or locked up particularly when there are inquisitive young toddlers in the house. Many commercial agents are now available for use as satisfactory antiseptics and when used according to the directions that come with them are both effective in inhibiting the formation of ammonia and safe to use.

The commercial diaper services use these agents but only with extreme caution and care, for like any antiseptic, they can be harmful when employed in excessive or toxic amounts. (Remember that poisons can be absorbed into the body through normal unbroken skins— and even more easily, through the raw open surfaces that are often present with a diaper rash.) If diapers are laundered at home, it would be advisable for the mother to consult with her physician before using any antiseptic agents.

When we come right down to it, strict cleanliness and complete sterility of the diapers (such as diaper services insist on) is the best prevention of diaper rash.

Treatment of the uncomplicated (i.e. non-infected) rash should employ only simple and painless methods. First, of course, is the removal of the diaper as soon as it has become soiled. This is followed by cleansing the involved skin and drying it. In those instances in which the area is raw, soap and water may prove irritating as well as painful and a soap substitute or a bland oil such as baby oil is recommended. Exposure of the parts to air and sun or, when this is not possible, exposure to the heat of an ordinary electric light bulb will aid in the healing of the skin. Many healing ointments, salves, powders, etc., are commercially available and are effective methods of treatment. If the rash does not respond to treatment, or appears to be getting worse, consult your physician, as an infected diaper rash can lead to serious trouble. Don't experiment with your baby—and don't accept your well-meaning neighbor's advice.

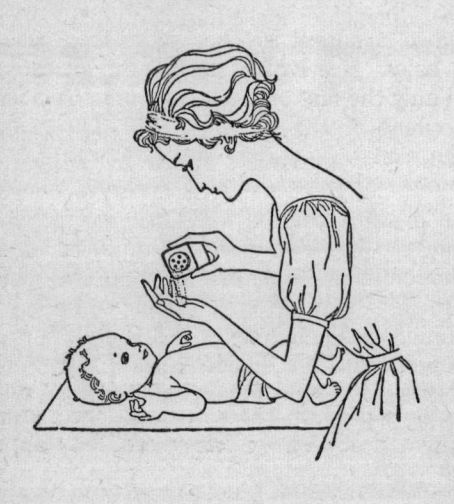

Care of Baby's Skin

by H. Laurence Dowd, M.D.

WHAT is a baby's greatest attraction? Many people think it is the eyes. But after the eyes comes a baby's skin, which should have a good healthy tinge whether the infant is breast or bottle fed. A baby's skin should be elastic, free from any eruption, with a smooth, creamy feel, and should be neither hot nor dry.

Rough skin and rashes, particularly in infants, may be due to a deficiency or an excess of some nutrient. There is no one food that is apt to cause such a condition, consequently the diet of the individual baby should be checked to be sure it isn't out of balance. I once saw a nursing baby's face which was a mass of blotches. I prescribed only the first of the breast milk, thus reducing the fat content of the diet, and the skin cleared up quickly. Another baby on the bottle was getting an excessive amount of sugar. Its skin was red, blotchy and sensitive. The skin became clear when the sugar was reduced to proper proportions.

Normal everyday care of a baby's skin, taking advantage of the many fine products designed for this purpose, should keep it healthy and rash-free. Baby oil, lotion, powder and soap are all easily available and inexpensive, and when used as recommended by your own doctor, can help prevent diaper rash and other eruptions. Occasionally a heat rash or diaper rash may appear, or the baby's skin may look red or chafed. Once such a condition has been cleared up, efforts should be made by the mother to prevent a recurrence. Strict cleanliness and the judicious use of gentle soap and other baby cosmetics at bath time and at diaper changes will work wonders in keeping your infant's skin healthy.

Mothers become worried and nervous when they see a baby's skin breaking out, but the rash can usually be banished quickly with proper care. Your pediatrician will tell you what to use to clear up the child's skin and to prevent a recurrence of the rash.

Of course, certain skin diseases may occur in infancy and childhood. For instance, edema or swelling of the skin has a large number of causes in infancy, chiefly from disturbances of the kidneys, stomach and bowels, from general debilitation, from a wrong diet (particularly one with an excessive amount of starch), and as a result of certain diseases, such as erysipelas, and severe pertussis (whooping-cough). Urticaria (hives) also may occur. They may be of an hereditary nature or related to the diet, and may be very troublesome and persistent.

Erythema, a localized redness in small or large areas with no elevation of the skin, and perhaps moderate burning or itching, results from over-exposure to the sun's rays, to heat or cold, to medicines or chemical substances, or as a result of the injection of certain drugs. Chafing or severe erythema is fairly common, not infrequently passing into an eczema, the result of friction between two moist surfaces, or from the continued contact of soiled diapers. Fatness of the baby, warm weather, allergies, and carelessness in diapering are predisposing causes.

If a drug or special medication produces a skin reaction in your baby, don't try to treat it without consulting your doctor. This may happen as a result of "wonder drugs" such as sulfa or the antibiotics, but it may also be caused by other medicines. It is always wise

CARE OF BABY'S SKIN

to check a baby's condition regularly after any drug has been given. One practice doctors constantly warn mothers against is re-dosing a baby with a drug that was prescribed for one illness when similar symptoms appear.

It is also possible for a drug to affect the infant through the milk of the mother. Chloral may cause a scarletinal eruption, or one of some other nature. The iodides give rise often to an acne-like eruption; less frequently to other rashes. Phenolphthalein can produce an urticarial eruption. The injection of sera, such as diphtheria antitoxin, may be followed by urticaria or an eruption resembling erythema multiforme, or of a type resembling scarlet fever or rubella (German measles), from the fifth to the ninth day after injection. Usually a rise of temperature and articular pain accompany the rash. Mothers should keep a close watch over their babies after injections or medications have been given; one baby will show no reaction at all, while another may. Call your doctor immediately if any change takes place in your baby's appearance.

To soothe and heal severe skin conditions, zinc oxide is a proven remedy, and when combined with lanolin, is a satisfactory preparation. Ask your druggist for one with a faint aroma, and one that will not deteriorate. Occasionally, you may have to treat abrasions, chafed and chapped skin, small cuts or fissures and minor skin irritations. A good treatment is wet dressings saturated with a solution of boric acid, or a medicated antiseptic cream for the acute stage; then regular applications of a good baby cream. But you should check your pediatrician if the skin stays hot or dry, and your treatment is not quickly effective.

Since diaper rash is the most frequently seen of the various rashes, every mother should know how to treat it effectively. Your doctor will advise you which of the many baby products to use when and if it appears.

The Art of Mothering

by **Dorothy V. Whipple, M.D.**

WHEN all of the mountains of scientific knowledge about babies and mothers are sifted through, we come up with one simple and fundamental fact. The mother who truly loves her baby and has self-respect and confidence in herself has powerful instincts to guide her. There is not one right way to care for a baby. Each mother finds her own technique. But she gets across her attitude—and this is what lays the foundation for personality for years to come.

Motherhood carries responsibilities that will go on for a decade or two, 24 hours a day, 365 days a year. Some mothers will do the entire job themselves, single-handed—others will delegate some of it—but the responsibility can never be delegated. Working mothers as well as mothers who stay home—they both have the same responsibilities toward their children. A great deal is known these days about babies and how they grow—what is good for them—what is not good for them. It is the basis for this knowledge we bring you here—to make motherhood a joy for you instead of a worry.

Be a relaxed mother. A baby is at peace, sleeps and eats like an angel if his mother is calm, confident and free from tensions. No baby likes a worried, nervous, jittery person. He may not understand words but he has an

THE ART OF MOTHERING

uncanny abiilty to absorb a mother's state of mind. If a mother's arms are jerky and tense as she picks up her baby; if her voice is shrill, the baby objects. He cries, refuses to eat, sleeps fitfully. A baby thrives if the emotional climate is calm, loving and warm, regardless of the exact techniques used in his care. He objects vociferously to nervous tension no matter how scientifically he is cared for.

Tricks of mother's trade. While the general attitude is important, there are tricks to baby care that can help. But remember they are *just* tricks—what is truly important is what is deep down inside the mother.

Holding your baby. Learn how to hold your baby. A newborn is floppy. He cannot hold his head up nor support his back. Be sure to put your hand at his neck when you pick him up and give his back support.

Swaddle him well. A newborn is more comfortable and he sleeps more peacefully, when wrapped up snugly in a blanket. Up to the very moment of birth, he knew nothing but a very confined space. It takes time to get accustomed to a wide open world.

Care for his skin. A baby's skin is thin and delicate. Use soap sparingly when you bathe him or sponge him off. Keep him warm but not overwarm. Wash his bottom gently with clear water when you change his diaper and apply a small amount of either baby powder or oil. If he gets a little rash in the diaper area—and such rashes are very common—leave his diaper off and expose his skin to the fresh air.

Cuddle him often. Baby likes soft sounds and gentle stroking. He likes good warm milk when he is hungry and a comfortable place to sleep when all of his needs are met. He does not like bright lights, loud noises, pain, hunger or jittery people. He likes the security of his mother's arms and the loving sounds her voice makes when she picks him up and feeds him.

Bathing a baby. This is a simple operation and it doesn't take a professional nurse to do it well. The object is to get the baby clean in such a way that he is neither chilled nor frightened nor hurt. Any loving mother can bathe her baby successfully.

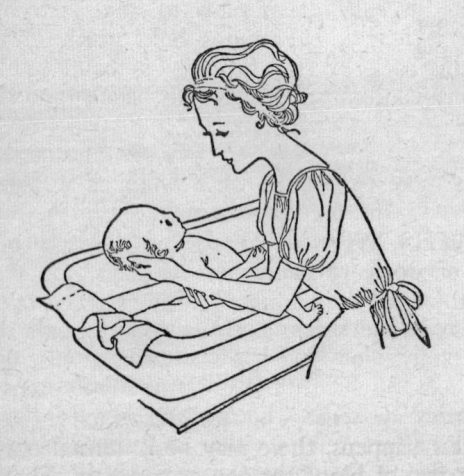

At Home With Baby

by **Herbert M. Porter, M.D.**

EVERY pediatrician is accustomed to frantic calls from new mothers who are suffering a severe case of stage fright on finding themselves alone at home with a new baby. This is understandable but it is also unnecessary. Practice makes perfect in baby care as in everything else, and the sooner a mother learns to know her newborn, the quicker she becomes professional and relaxed about his care. Here is some basic advice that should banish those quaking fears about handling a new baby.

BATHS. When to start giving the baby baths is a source of worry to many new mothers. Do not bathe your baby until the umbilical cord has fallen off and the navel has healed. Instead, cleanse him once a day with a good baby lotion. Clean the base of the umbilical cord with a cotton swab soaked in alcohol to hasten the drying process and speed up the falling off of the cord. After this happens, there may be a normal oozing of a drop or two of blood for one or two days. Fecal matter which is stuck to the skin can be removed with a little warm baby oil.

If the baby has been circumcised, a little petroleum jelly placed around the incised edges of the penis will keep it from sticking to the diaper. Do not bathe him until the circumcision is healed. This takes about a week.

CRYING. When the baby cries, mothers get panicky and jump to the conclusion that he is hungry. The thing to do is find out why he is crying.

He may be lying in an uncomfortable position or be tangled up in his blanket. If so, he will probably stop crying when you pick him up and resettle him. He may be wet or lying in a soiled diaper. If so, change the diaper. Some infants are apparently more fastidious than others and object to lying in a wet or soiled diaper; some do not complain. Knowing your baby, you will know if this is what is making him cry. He may be too cold or too warm. Adjust the blankets accordingly and make the room warmer or cooler as indicated.

If none of these situations appears to be the cause of his crying, then consider whether he is hungry. Here you need to think about what took place at his last previous feeding. If that feeding was at least 3½ hours earlier, he is probably hungry, and it is time to feed him again. If, however, he had his meal about 2 hours ago and took his entire feeding, then it is extremely unlikely that he is crying from hunger. Look for another reason, perhaps a bubble of gas; try picking him up and burping him. Then put him right back in his crib. He will probably go to sleep immediately. But if he had his last meal 2 hours ago and only took part of it, then he is probably hungry. In such a situation, give the baby water or weak tea to tide him over until the next feeding.

Finally, the baby may be crying because he has slept enough and wants to play. Remember that his moods and needs do not remain the same.

FORMULA. Before you left the hospital, your doctor probably gave you a formula, either one of the new ready-prepared types, already bottled and ready to give the baby without warming—or one that you would have to prepare. If it was the latter, you were undoubtedly told how to prepare it. As your infant grows, your doctor will tell you when and how to increase or change the formula.

In giving the bottle, make certain that the infant's lips are well up on the bulbous part of the nipple. This part acts as a seal and prevents air from entering his mouth as he sucks. Do not under any circumstances let the baby lie flat with the bottle propped up by a pillow, blanket or some propping device.

Make certain that the milk is not flowing too quickly or too slowly. The flow is right if the milk just drips out when you hold the full bottle upside down and give it a gentle shake. If the milk flows too quickly, the baby may choke; if it flows too slowly, he will work too hard and get tired before he has had his full feeding. If the flow is too fast, the formula may be too hot, the collar around the bottle may be too loose, or the nipple may be worn out (and should be discarded). If the flow is too slow, the opening of the nipple may be clogged or the collar is too tight. Nipples last about three or four weeks. They should be replaced after this time. The pre-filled nursers are disposable and you have a new nipple each time you use one.

BURPING THE BABY. How and when and why to burp (or bubble) the baby is as important as how and when to feed him.

When an infant cries, breathes, sucks, or swallows, he takes in air. It is normal for him to have some air (gas) in his stomach and intestines, but an excessive amount makes him very uncomfortable. To help the infant get rid of the excessive gas, hold him against your chest or support him in a sitting position and gently pat him on the back.

Many mothers complain that it is difficult to bubble the baby. Don't make a complicated ritual out of a simple procedure. If the baby doesn't burp within five minutes, prop him up in a semi-reclining position for ten minutes and then try again. If he still doesn't bubble, put him to sleep on his right side or on his stomach. These positions are helpful because they allow the air to rise above the milk in the stomach.

SPITTING UP. Spitting up after a meal is the result of the milk in the stomach being forced back into the esophagus and then appearing in the mouth. If a baby is bottle fed and spits up frequently, check the flow and temperature of the milk. Make certain that you are burping him well and that you are not over-feeding him. Try propping him up for fifteen minutes after each feeding. If spitting continues, check your doctor.

WATER. Doctors are often asked how much water the baby should drink. There is no hard and fast answer. As infant's requirements for water are normally met by an adequate formula, and he may not want additional water. But it is often offered between feedings as a temporizing measure. Some infants drink very little extra water; others will drink it only when it is slightly sweetened with sugar; still others drink several ounces a day.

VITAMINS. Another question that mothers often ask concerns vitamins. These will be prescribed by your doctor. Most babies are given vitamins A, C and D, starting in the second week.

BOWEL MOVEMENTS. This is always a problem to new mothers who worry about the infant's bowel movements. The type and frequency of the baby's stools depends upon the type of milk he is being fed. Breast fed infants have loose, golden yellow stools, while babies fed with formula usually have yellow, pasty stools. Breast fed infants usually have bowel movements more frequently than infants that are bottle fed. Stools may vary in number from six to eight daily to one every two to three days. They decrease in number as the baby grows.

Sound Sleep Habits

by **Dorothy V. Whipple, M.D.**

A young baby loves to sleep. Give him a chance and he will snooze away most of the hours of every day. As he gets a little older he will stay awake more and more. One of the objects of baby care is to arrange life so that the baby sleeps happily at night and confines his waking time to the daylight hours.

Soon after birth, a baby sleeps 18 to 20 hours out of the 24; by three months he has cut his sleep down to 16 to 18 hours; by six months to 14 to 16 hours. By the time he is a year old, 12 to 14 hours is usually enough.

The newborn wakes up at intervals during the 24 hours; he doesn't know anything about day and night. His inside barometer is not tuned to the sun. Take care of his needs as they arise; love him, hold him, feed him when he asks for you. As soon as he has everything he needs, he will go back to sleep. During the early weeks a baby is apt to be noisy when he sleeps. He grunts and growls and snorts. This is usual and normal; don't worry about it.

A month-old baby will begin to take one long sleep of 6 to 8 hours. It's amazing how many babies, all on their own, choose the night for this long sleep. However, it's a good idea to help a baby make this decision. Don't let your infant sleep more than four hours in the daytime. If he is fast asleep at the end of four hours, wake him up, disturb him. He will not be awake long before he discovers it would be nice to eat. A baby must get his quota of milk. He may be able to manage on 5 feedings in 24 hours, but if he skips one in the day he's sure to want it at night. Try to persuade him to eat at not less than 4 hour intervals during the day, then let him sleep as long as he will nights.

A baby grows up to enjoy regularity. As he gets a little older, he will set a schedule for himself. But he is quite amenable to adapting his schedule to yours. Try to start the day at the same hour every day. Wake the baby up at this time, if necessary; then each day will slip into the same pattern.

At three months of age, the baby will want to stay awake longer between feedings. Let him spend his waking hours outside of his crib—a playpen is the safest spot. Then, when it is sleeping time, back to his crib. In this way he becomes accustomed to going to sleep when he is put in his crib.

Babies are individuals right from the beginning. Some need more sleep than others. Some babies like to sleep right after a meal, others feel sociable when their stomachs are full. Your baby will be a happy baby if you take his individuality into account.

But while each baby has his own personality, there are a few universal characteristics. All babies object to tension, anxiety and nervousness. A baby seems to know immediately if his mother is trying to rush him through a feeding; he knows if she is upset. He doesn't like tense arms and shrill voices. These things upset him; he cannot relax, he will not eat properly and his sleep will be disturbed.

It's good to remember that during the first year of life babies want to sleep. This is not always true of a little run-around who sometimes fights sleep because he hates to give up the fascinating world of play. But during the first year, very few babies fight sleep. However, some babies will cry when they are sleepy. If he is put in his crib, his crying soon ceases and he goes to sleep.

Nowadays there is so much talk about the evil effects of letting a baby "cry it out" that sometimes a young mother is afraid to put a crying baby in his crib, and she actually keeps him awake by her attentions. True, long periods of yelling are to be avoided, but a few minutes of crying before sleep may be the way your baby adjusts to life. Most babies cry to be picked up but some of them *do* cry to be put down.

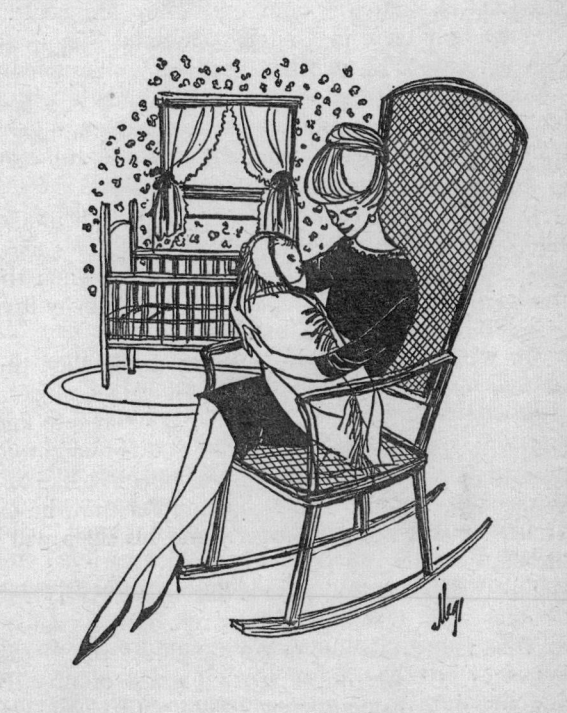

Colic and the Nervous Baby

by Helen Evans Reid, M.D.

MODERN babies seldom cry. They are healthier than they were in Granny's day, and they are infinitely better fed. The clothes they wear are designed for comfort, freedom from restraint and warmth without weight. Their mothers are capable, and baby equipment and furniture is more efficient, sanitary and functional than ever before. Occasionally, though, one hears of a healthy baby who raises his small voice in complaint, who expresses his discomfort vocally to the great distress and concern of his parents. A short crying spell, relieved by feeding, changing or cuddling, is, of course, of no significance. But the very small infant who, in the first three months, wakes up crying and struggling, about an hour after each feeding, probably has colic.

So common is colic in small infants that some authorities regard it as normal and feel that all babies have it in more or less degree at some time or another in the first few months of life. This may be an exaggeration. Certainly there is great variation among babies, from the one who experiences only an occasional attack to the unhappy wee mite who seems to suffer after every feeding.

Colic, though common, is exceedingly distressing to the child and to the mother. In a typical attack, the baby will awake from sleep with a screaming cry. His pain is obviously severe and acute for his crying is quite unlike that by which he indicates other discomforts or hunger. The legs are drawn up stiffly over the abdomen which often seems hard and distended. The screaming usually ends suddenly with passage of gas by the bowel, and the exhausted baby falls back to sleep. The length of the attack may vary from a few minutes to more than an hour. Late afternoon and evening seem the worst times of day.

What causes colic? Probably several factors. The actual pain seems due to distension of the bowel with the gas which the child seems unable to pass along. To some extent, the nature of the feeding may produce this situation. But changing and altering the formula is usually of little help. It may be that the newborn human infant is not so completely "ripe" as other newborns of other species, and the nerves controlling the bowels are not mature enough to function to perfection until about three months of age. Very rarely, a true allergy to milk may be the cause. And doctors and psychologists are still looking for other causes such as emotional factors, relationship to the mother, etc.

So distressing is the attack that almost any means that will give relief to the baby are justified. Mothers have found that placing the baby face down over the knee or on a warm hot water bottle, or gently rubbing the abdomen will help the baby to expel the gas. Sometimes a drink of warm water or a feeding will stimulate the bowels sufficiently and achieve the same result. An enema will usually help. By all means, pick up the baby. Cuddle him warmly, placing him against your shoulder.

How can you prevent colic? Discuss your baby's feedings with your doctor to be sure that quality and quantity are right. For the bottle fed baby, see that the holes in the nipples are neither so large that the feeding comes through too rapidly, causing him to gulp air, nor so small that the feeding comes slowly, permitting him to feed overlong and perhaps, to suck air. Be sure "he says his bubble" or burps two or three times during each feeding.

Even with the utmost care, you may not be able to prevent all attacks, but he will thrive in spite of his distress and no permanent harm will result from colic. Do what you can each time to relieve it and take heart. Babies grow out of colic.

Occasionally too, we see the nervous high-strung baby who seems to cry all the time. He is a little bundle of nerves, is tense and worried looking, holds his legs and arms stiffly, cries loudly and long, and is roused from his fitful slumbers by the slightest sound. He is known as the "hypertonic baby" whose muscles seem so taut that relaxation is impossible.

There isn't much you can do to change his nature. He will grow out of a good deal of the stiffness as his nervous system matures, but he is likely to become the intense driving adult, impatient of frustrations and ulcer-prone—the executive type.

He needs extra food for he uses up a lot of energy, and his formula must be adjusted to provide it, along with more solids. He reacts vocally and physically to his feelings of hunger and even when they are satisfied, he cannot let go enough to relax in drowsy contentment. So while he is tiny he is better on a flexible feeding schedule.

The nervous baby requires more cuddling and more quiet. A calm, unhurried mother is an asset though the very irritability of the baby makes it almost impossible for her to remain placid. If she can manage it, he should be handled with slow, sure movements, to avoid startling or exciting him. The baby's doctor can be a great help with this child for he can prescribe safe, non-habit-forming sedatives which will promote relaxation and induce sleep. While they are safe, if controlled carefully, these drugs should only be given under the strictest medical supervision so that they do not build up to harmful levels.

The high-strung child, treated with understanding and infinite patience and affection, can become a vivid and sparkling personality, talented and energetic, though he will probaby always be "the nervous type." If his energies are guided and directed properly, he will become an effective adult.

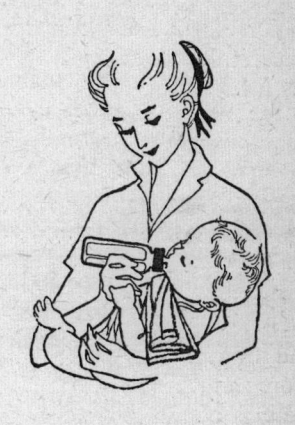

Making a Feeding Schedule

by **Alfred J. Vignec, M.D.**

THE issue of self-demand has caused many heated discussions in medical and psychological circles for some years now. Actually, in its broader aspects, it represents far more than a method of feeding. If the principle of self-demand is truly carried out in handling a baby or small child, it becomes a basic method of child rearing. The question is, can this method work and is it a wise approach or, used indiscriminately, can it give rise to more problems than it solves?

It is well to remember that patterns of child management tend to run in cycles. Without wanting to inject a flippant note, fashions in child care can be as varied as those in women's clothing. The pendulum tends to swing from one extreme to the other. I say this primarily because in the period just before self-demand came into favor an entirely different system was in popular use and had many enthusiastic exponents. The child was not to be picked up or fondled, was to be handled with detachment, was to be left to cry, taught to adhere rigidly to the schedules prescribed by adults, etc. It seems difficult to believe that people actually followed these stern policies and were just as convinced that their behavior towards the infant and small child was correct as we are today.

There is no question that the stern, cold disciplinary measures of this period were incorrect from a psychological viewpoint. The child was often lonely, and felt unloved. Many basic insecurities were directly traceable to the lack of displayed parental affection, although doubtless parents were quite fond of their children as they are today. Self-demand in its inception was a form of rebellion against this method of handling.

Let us first examine what is meant by "self-demand." It means initially that the infant regulates his own feeding program. If practiced in the extreme, the infant is fed whenever he cries, once it is determined that there is no other apparent reason for his distress (such as wet or soiled diapers, open safety pins, etc.) This system was practiced on formula-fed as well as breast-fed infants. Later, when solid feedings were introduced, the infant was permitted considerable latitude in his choices concerning amount and kind of food accepted, and also in some cases with regard to number of feedings—although by this time some effort was usually made by the pediatrician to establish a basic regime, as too many solid feedings could cause difficulty.

However, self-demand, if truly practiced, did not stop with feeding. It extended also into the fields of toilet training, sleep patterns, and most of all, general behavior. The true exponent of self-demand believed that the infant should always be picked up when he cried. The toddler and small child was permitted to express himself with complete freedom in his games and other activities. The adult was held responsible for the removal of dangerous and forbidden articles from the child's environment. Restrictive punishment of any kind was frowned upon. Frustration was to be avoided. Toilet training was to be left to the child. Sleep patterns were regulated by the child.

This sounds like an ideal arrangement. Freedom is desired by all, young and old. An atmosphere without restraints is an enviable one. Unfortunately it is also an impossible one to attain. The world is not without restraints and from the moment of birth each of us is subjected to them in greater or lesser degree. Even diapers are a restriction imposed by civilized society. Certainly clothes are.

Self-demand in its extreme form is a contradiction to the basic principles of life. In this world there are no true non-conformists except criminals or deviants, and even these are bound by the very rules which they are attempting to break. Let us examine the effect of an extremely lax program on the child. He very rapidly comes to govern the household, rather than fit into it. This may not be the goal, but it is too often the outcome. To begin with, his habits of eating disrupt the family immediately. The mother is obliged to drop every thing and prepare odd quantities of formula at illogical hours or, as the case may be, breast feed. Not only does this create a hardship which may eventually be coupled with resentment, but it very often produces colic in the infant. Also, he may accept only an ounce or two at a time, because he had little or no actual desire to eat in the first place. Once on solids, new complications arise. Not infrequently the infant goes so far as to refuse all prepared foods so that the mother must resort to cooking and mashing fresh foods, and these too, may be rejected. Later on, the problems increase even more. It is the rare child indeed who induces and accomplishes its own toilet training program successfully and the rarer one who can wisely regulate his own hours of sleep. It is almost impossible in the modern apartment or home for the parent to remove all undersirable objects from the baby's reach, although certainly the greatest discretion must be used. But ask the mother of any family of two or more what her household would be like without the judicious use of "no-no" and "mustn't touch."

What, then, is the solution? Are we to return to the rigid disciplinary measures of our forebears and teach the child "frustration in the cradle"? Certainly not. As is the case with so many problems of successful living, the solution lies in the practice of moderation. By no means must the parents' guiding hand be withdrawn. The little tyrant who rules the home and shouts for his way, throws his dinner on the floor and gobbles sweets, stays up half the night, and is in constant danger of accident, is disobedient and unmanageable from the outset, is an unhappy child as well, and is often unpopular outside of the intimate family circle. The happy child, on the other hand, is the one who has learned not frustration, but how to conform.

The ideal feeding plan for the new baby is one which is set up by the mother and at the same time leaves latitude for the baby's preferences. If the infant prefers to eat at 1-5-9-1-5-9 instead of 2-6-10-2-6-10, there is no reason to deny him. All schedules should be planned plus or minus an hour, so that the baby who is due to eat at 6 may eat at any time between 5 and 7, when hungry. He should not be forced. He should be led in a fashion that will eventually make him an acceptable and accepted part of the family group. It is interesting to note that the behavior problems arising from an indiscreet use of the principles of self-demand usually occur far more frequently in first or only children than in later arrivals. This is undoubtedly because over-zealous effort on the mother's part interfered with her better judgment in the case of a first child. By the time the second arrived, her viewpoint was clearer.

As with feeding, other programs of child rearing should take into consideration the general pattern of the household, the child's preferences, and the child's eventual adjustment to strangers and society as a whole. It should be remembered that it is the child who is flexible, not the adult. This has been known for centuries. "As the twig is bent, so the tree is inclined" is an old proverb. It is proven beyond question that children grow gradually and successfully into widely varying patterns by the study of different societies. Children absorb the rules and customs of their separate worlds whether they be Eskimos, Chinese, Samoans, or Caucasians.

As the child grows older he should be helped to understand why certain demands are made of him. He should be given choices wherever possible, and quite freely—but there must be general rules to govern conduct, as we all have rules to live by. The child who is to set his own standards is as insecure due to lack of stability and guidance as the child who has been over-disciplined into frustration and loneliness. It must also be considered and remembered that children have an infinite variety of individual differences and it is wrong to curb these and attempt to cut every child to a given pattern. Even within a family, one child may have his bowel movements regularly and be happily trained as soon as he sits and stands freely. Another with more irregular habits may wait until much older and resist earlier efforts with determination and resentment. One may abandon the bottle early and delight in his cup—another become an inveterate finger sucker and refuse milk entirely if his bottle is removed.

The secret of a successful mother-child relationship and a happy childhood within the family and in the outer world lies not in any fixed set of rules. It is wise to avoid extremes and to rely on judgment and understanding. Understanding, above all other things, is the keynote as it is always, in all relationships throughout life.

The Premature Baby

by R. Cannon Eley, M.D.

AN infant born alive and weighing 5 pounds 8 ounces, or less, is considered a "premature" infant regardless of the duration of the period of pregnancy. This definition has, for practical purposes, been accepted by the medical profession although it is known that certain elements such as sex, race, multiple births and the health of the mother during pregnancy may be influencing factors. These infants are divided into four groups according to their respective weights and it naturally follows that the smaller the infant, the poorer are its chances for survival. It is also obvious that because of their small size they are subject to disturbances that may endanger their life and which are not encountered in normal full-term babies who have more resistance to infections. For this reason most hospitals have a special nursery staffed by nurses and doctors who have had special training in the care of such small infants, and who are fully aware of their problems and dangers.

There are several principles concerned in the care of premature infants such as (1) maintenance of normal body temperature (2) maintenance of adequate nutritional requirements (3) prevention of infection (4) constant and intelligent nursing care.

Immediately after birth the baby is placed in a heated crib or incubator which has previously been prepared in anticipation of the birth. A quick, yet careful, physical examination should be made at this time provided the infant's general condition permits it. Care should be taken not to over-expose, or handle, the newcomer and all of this should be done with the patient in the incubator. A physician experienced in the care of prematures can make such an examination in a surprisingly short period of time and without danger to the infant. For the same reasons the initial cleansing of the skin etc., should be omitted at this time and performed later, when the progress of the baby has proven to be satisfactory.

There is no immediate hurry about starting feedings; in fact, it is considered best to withhold any feeding by mouth for at least 24 to 48 hours. When feedings are begun it is usually with a weak solution rather than breast milk or some modified form of cow's milk. This solution is better tolerated and less apt to cause vomiting. The method of feeding, i.e., by bottle, dropper, or by a tube that may be passed through the nose to the stomach, will depend on the size, weight, vigor and activity of the baby. Often some of these prematures have such a poor sucking reflex (mechanism) that bottle feeding with a nipple or even with a dropper is out of the question. In these babies it may be necessary to have a surgeon operate so that milk can be introduced directly into the stomach. The amount given at a single feeding and the frequency of feedings vary with the weight and general condition of the individual baby and as the infant shows satisfactory progress the amount of breast milk or the strength of the formula is gradually increased to meet the nutritional, i.e., fat, carbohydrate, protein and calorie requirements. Vitamins and iron requirements are usually introduced about the second or third week of life.

Prevention of infection among premature infants is of more importance than it is with full-term babies, as the former group have no immunity, are more vulnerable, and are more susceptible. To minimize the possibility of infections, the exclusion of visitors, removal of personnel who may or who do have an infection, the use of mask (mouth and nose), cap and gown, and the scrupulous cleansing of hands are mandatory in any well organized premature nursery. And, needless to say, any baby who develops an infection should be removed from the nursery at once.

Nursery care cannot be stressed too much. It must be constant and intelligent by nurses especially trained in the field of the care of these newborns. An alert nurse will detect unfavorable signs and symptoms at their beginning and notify the physician responsible for the care of the baby. This may not only prevent a serious complication, but at times save a life. Thus it is not only the maintenance of temperature and proper oxygen concentration in the incubator and expert technique in feeding these "premies," but the constant alertness for vital signs that are the responsibilities of a well-trained and conscientious nurse.

And now we take our baby—no longer a "premie" —home. When the baby's weight is satisfactory, discharge is permissible. The youngster is gaining regularly, taking his feedings well, is active and usually causing no concern except to the parents, who understandably are a bit on the anxious side! However, their physician plus the expert advice of the community visiting nurse will see them "over the hump." It is important, just as it was in the hospital, to take all measures to avoid and prevent infections of any type even now.

(PKU) Phenylketonuria

by R. Cannon Eley, M.D.

OVER thirty years ago a new hereditary disease became recognized and since then has been known as "phenylketonuria" or PKU. At first thought to be a clearcut single entity, it was soon recognized as possessing a wide range of disorders with both typical and atypical manifestations. The former is a grave and serious situation resulting in damage to the brain, thereby producing mental retardation. This form requires treatment, whereas the atypical types are harmless and, therefore, treatment is not indicated. This disturbance, PKU, is due to the presence of an acid known as phenylalanine (which is present in foods containing protein) in abnormally high amounts in the blood. It is the result of a genetic defect.

The genetic defect lies in the inability of the individual to produce a specific enzyme in the liver, thereby making it impossible to convert phenylalanine, a "toxic" substance, into a harmless acid known as tyrosine. There then follows a rapid accumulation of phenylalanine in the blood and its appearance in the urine as phenylpyruvic acid. There is still some confusion as to which of these two acids is responsible for the brain damage of the infant, as both children and adults have been shown to have abnormal amounts of phenylalanine in their blood yet are perfectly normal both mentally and physically. As

PKU (PHENYLKETONURIA)

newer and more refined methods of diagnosis have been developed, it is now thought that PKU occurs once in every 10,000 births rather than once in every 20,000 as was previously estimated. As the hereditary trait is a recessive one, it does not necessarily follow that all the children of "carrier" parents may have the disease, but rather one in four.

If the disorder is not recognized early in life (i.e. the first 3—4 months) but is allowed to progress, damage to the brain occurs and is of an irreversible nature. Associated with mental retardation, other manifestations may appear such as convulsion, skin discoloration, random and purposeless movements of the extremities, spastic muscles, and a type of eczema that is resistant to treatment. Characteristically these infants are blue-eyed and blond. Early diagnosis and the prompt introduction of carefully controlled and supervised treatment are essential if progression of the disease and increased brain damage is to be halted.

Up to this point we have assumed that the manifestations of PKU were the result of the inability of the infant per se to digest his protein-containing foods in a normal manner. But what about maternal PKU and its possible effect on the baby before birth? It is well known that during the last month or two of intrauterine life, the brain develops at a remarkable rate of growth and is readily susceptible to agents that may be harmful to it. Since 1963 there has been accumulating increasing evidence that infants without the disease born of mothers with the disease may be mentally retarded. The high incidence of this affliction among these babies has raised the question as to whether or not the high level of phenylalanine in the mother's circulation may not have damaged the brain prior to birth. If this is proven to be true, would it not be advisable to test all pregnant women for the presence of PKU? Even more to the point, should not such tests be performed on all specimens of blood obtained for premarital examination? In this manner, unsuspected or unrecognized individuals of apparent normal or near normal intelligence would be detected and the risk of having a normal baby at the termination of pregnancy be known to them. This poses many pertinent questions; personal, legal, public health-wise as well as religious. It is certainly one aspect of PKU that should be explored and clarified.

As previously stated, the presence of phenylalanine in excessive amounts in the blood results from the inability of the body to properly utilize foods containing protein. Since the newborn seldom receives breast milk (which contains less protein than cow's milk) or a formula before the second or third day of life, tests for the presence of phenylpyruvic acid in the urine are of no diagnostic value until after protein has been ingested. Therefore, diagnostic tests are not in order until between the 3rd—4th to 7th day of life. So called "screening" tests are available for all newborn infants and are now employed in practically all maternity hospitals prior to the discharge of the baby, as well as in doctor's offices for either initial examinations or for repeat examinations. One of these is a simple procedure and consists of the addition of a few drops of ferric chloride to a fresh specimen of urine, or applying drops to a urine-soaked diaper, and watching for the presence or absence of the development of a blue color. Another test known as the "Gunthire Test" is performed on a drop of blood obtained from the infant's heel and allowed to dry on a piece of special filter paper. Even if these initial tests are negative, they should be repeated at 4 to 6 weeks of age. That they should be repeated on any infant born to a family that already has a child with PKU hardly needs to be stressed. To confirm the diagnosis, accurate levels of phenylalanine in the blood should be determined, for in this way only can errors in the diagnosis of true, typical cases of PKU be avoided. Although these tests are not mandatory in all states, many states have made them so.

PKU (PHENYLKETONURIA)

Treatment consists in the early introduction of, and strict adherence to a diet consisting of foods of low protein content. The diet is not a very palatable one and although it can usually be maintained without difficulty with the infant who is formula fed, adherence to it at a later date when the "toddler" or "run-about" can forage for himself offers a real problem. Although the therapeutic value of a diet low in phenylalanine has not yet been proven and has its proponents as well as its opponents, it is the only form of treatment now available and should be employed until better methods have been developed.

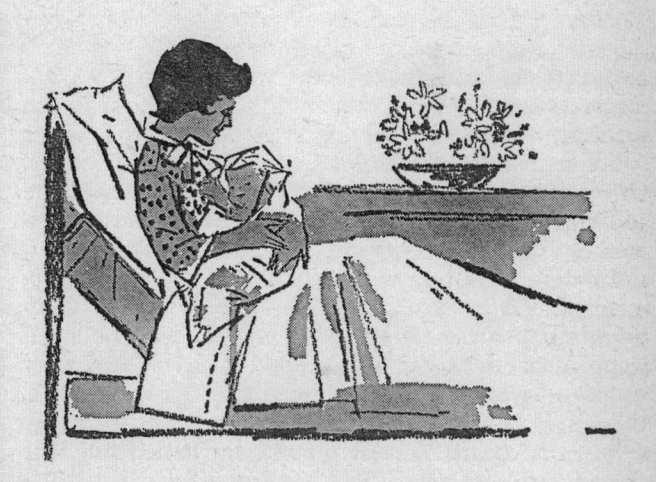

SECTION III

As the Baby Grows

Common Infections

by R. Cannon Eley, M.D.

THE arrival of fall and winter months usually heralds the beginning of seasonal infections among infants and children which are largely respiratory in nature. Thus the anxiousness and apprehension of parents at this period of the year is understandable. Many factors are responsible for the presence, as well as for the frequency of these illnesses. During the cold months there is much less outdoor activity, with the result that members of a family spend most of their time within the home and are more intimately in contact with each other. This, in turn, facilitates the transference of bacterial or viral infection from one member of the family to the other. Ventilation is likewise reduced and higher concentrations of infective agents are present in the homes. Similar conditions exist in the schools and children in attendance quite often contract some infection which does not make them sick, but which, when transmitted to a younger member of the family, such as a baby, may result in the "common cold" or a severe illness such as pneumonia. We all have witnessed the greater frequency of respiratory disease in the home where there are very young infants or children who have older sisters or brothers attending schools.

This introduces the question of the role of age on this frequency, and the course of infection. Immediately after birth certain bacterial infections which usually cause little if any trouble are particularly prevalent among newborn infants, whereas the more severe infections resulting from other bacterial invasions of the body such as the streptococcus germ, are more common during the latter part of infancy and early childhood. Yet in both situations the germs usually gain entrance to the body through the respiratory passages, the skin, or through the intestinal route. Thus the serious complications (morbidity) as well as the death rate (mortality) vary with age, being highest immediately after birth and gradually dropping and reaching their lowest points between the ages of 5 and 10 years. Part of this is due to changes caused by growth and development and, of course, to the development of immunity, i.e., protection by frequent exposure and contraction of minor forms of illness due to bacterial or viral agents. Early in life a baby may develop pneumonia from a certain germ whereas later in life this same "bug" may cause only a mild cold, cough, or bronchitis. Other conditions which may influence the frequency or severity of an illness are poor nutritional health as the direct result of an inadequate diet (fortunately rare in the United States), chronic illness such as tuberculosis, diabetes, heart disease, etc., and, of course, inadequate and poor housing conditions associated with low socio-economical conditions. With these predisposing factors in mind, let's consider some of the common infections of the season under discussion.

First, the viral group deserves attention as these agents are by far the commonest cause of the so-called cold or respiratory infection, as well as more severe infections such as severe chest pain, bronchitis, bronciolitis, pneumonia, or earaches and conjunctivitis (inflammation of the membranes protecting the eyes—"runny eyes"). Several separate groups of these agents exist, such as the "A-P-C" group, so-called because they cause infection of the adenoids, the pharynx, and the eyes. Then there are the Echo and Coxsacki groups—and so on down the line! Each member of each group usually has a number for its identification to distinguish it from other members, and at the same time to indicate the particular illness or trouble it may cause, such as croup, bronchitis, pneumonia, etc. There appears to be no end to the number of these agents, and almost each month new ones are being discovered and new diseases assigned to them. Many of the diseases for which the medical profession did not know the cause are now being recognized as caused by these viruses. At the present time treatment of these infections is purely "symptomatic," i.e., directed at the relief of pain, cough, reducing the temperature and where possible the prevention of complications. This can usually be accomplished by simple forms of medicine, proper rest and diet, and adequate fluid intake since the "magic drugs" have not proven to be helpful in any of these virus-produced infections. In fact, in some situations they may make matters worse.

Vaccines have proven helpful in the prevention of some of these infections among adults and particularly so in military training camps, but have not been helpful for patients of the pediatric age group.

Measles, a viral infection, occurs more frequently in late winter and early spring, but this disease need not occur as there are now vaccines that will prevent it, provided parents will take the time and effort to see that their children are immunized.

Certain diseases caused by bacteria are also more common during the fall and winter months than at any other period of the year. For example, streptococcal sore throat or tonsillitis, acutely infected and draining ears with or without complicating mastoiditis, and rheumatic fever. In previous years, these and similar infections from other germs which were so serious and so often accompanied by a high mortality rate, struck fear not only into the hearts of parents, but of nurses and doctors as well. Today the "miracle drugs" have greatly reduced, but not entirely eliminated, this danger. Diphtheria is known to be a disease of the winter months, but here again its occurrence may be said to be inexcusable as *it can be* prevented by immunization.

Meningitis may be caused by a virus, a parasite, or by bacteria. However, in the vast majority of instances, it is the result of a bacterial invasion of the brain. Crowded living quarters with the resulting close contacts of individuals is one of the most common causes of its spread. With the exception of one type (Epidemic or Meningococcal Meningitis) this form of disease was practically 100% fatal and even those patients who recovered suffered from such severe brain damage that they were useless to themselves and to society. Today the very opposite situation exists as few deaths and few complications occur provided an early diagnosis is made and treatment with appropriate "miracle drugs" is begun. These agents or drugs have proven to be very effective but have to be carefully chosen as some are more effective in some types of meningitis than others. Again early diagnosis and wise and prompt treatment can prove effective and equally, time delay can prove fatal.

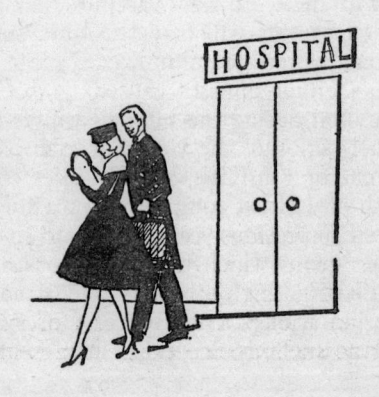

Colds

by **Dorothy V. Whipple, M.D.**

ALL little children have colds—some more than others—but the small child who does not have an occasional runny nose is very rare indeed.

As people grow older, the frequency of their colds decreases. School age children have fewer colds than toddlers and most grownups suffer only now and then from a cold.

The common cold is caused by a virus; however, there are perhaps 40 to 50 different viruses that can cause what we call a cold. Each attack leaves in its wake some immunity, but the immunity is only to the particular virus that caused that special cold. The child may come down next week with an illness that seems like the first one, but it is probably due to another virus. By the end of the first decade of life, most children have come in contact with the common viruses in their community, have built up some immunity to these organisms, and hence do not develop symptoms on subsequent encounters with these viruses.

We cannot today prevent colds as we are able to prevent measles, diphtheria, whooping cough and a host of serious diseases that in times past played havoc with the health of children. Someday we may have a single vaccine against the multitude of viruses causing colds, but no such vaccine exists at present. It is to be hoped that in the future even the common cold may be in the realm of almost forgotten diseases.

Good nutrition is a worthwhile goal in and of itself. Well nourished youngsters, however, as well as poorly nourished ones, succumb to colds. If a child's diet is good and he is getting his full quota of all the nutrients that make strong healthy bodies, his resistance to colds will not be increased by extra vitamins. A well nourished child, however, may recover more quickly than a poorly nourished one from any illness.

Children catch cold by coming in contact with a virus, almost always from the nose and throat of someone else. Wet feet and chilling do not cause colds. Viruses do not enter through the feet! There is nevertheless some relation between chilling and colds. Chilling causes a decreased blood flow through the blood vessels in the throat, setting up a transient local anemia. This means that a virus that happened to be present at this time has a greater chance of overcoming the natural defense mechanisms. The viruses that cause colds are present much of the time, ready to leap whenever defenses are down.

So the old adages "wear your rubbers", "put on a sweater when it's chilly", "don't sit in a draft", are still wise advice. It is also wise to get warmed up as soon as possible if you do get chilled, and while chilled, stay away from sniffly people.

Even when not chilled, toddlers pick up colds from each other. Health habits of little people between 2 and 4 years of age are conducive to the spread of nose and throat infections. A toddler is often inspired to hug a playmate, to breathe down his throat, to cough in his face. We teach youngsters not to do these things, but it takes time.

Reasonable precautions against colds are sensible but overprotection may do more harm than good. Toddlers need companionship of children their age. A few colds must be taken in stride, and hopefully each cold will leave some immunity that will pay future dividends.

The symptoms of a cold in a little child are runny nose, (at first a clear watery secretion, later a thick mucosy one), a little loss of appetite, irritability, a low fever (100-101°), sometimes some cough. A simple uncomplicated cold usually lasts about a week. There is no magic treatment for a cold. Antibiotics (either by injection or by mouth) do not help—viruses are not killed by these drugs. Antihistamines are sometimes harmful to a little child. These drugs dry up secretions in the nose and throat but do not kill the germs causing the illness. The germs may migrate into the deeper recesses of the chest where moisture is normally present, and if they get a chance to grow there, they may cause more serious illness, such as bronchitis or pneumonia. The best treatment of a simple cold is what is called symptomatic treatment, that is, make the child as comfortable as possible while his own defenses are curing him. He should be reasonably quiet so his energies can be used to fight his infection. If a youngster feels tired he may be quiet and happy in bed, but if he is eager to play, he may be much quieter if allowed out of bed with "quiet toys." He may eat what he wants of ordinary food, no special diet is required. Extra liquids to drink are helpful. A little aspirin will make him less fussy and irritable. A vaporizer with plain steam is soothing to irritated mucus membranes and eases a cough. The vaporizer is especially useful when secretions are thick. The warm steamy air keeps the secretions liquid and avoids the clogged nose that interferes with breathing and sucking. We want the runny nose to dry up, but we want it to dry up because the child is well, not because we have artificially dried it with drugs. As long as a child has a cold he is better off with a freely running nose. It is nature's response to the infection and a useful tool in recovery.

Nose drops, sprays, most drugs, do not really help a child get over a cold. The most that can be said for such measures is that they give the mother the sense that she is "doing something."

Little children suffer from other respiratory diseases besides colds. Some of these illnesses are more serious and need more treatment than a simple cold. While there is no absolute way for a mother to distinguish a simple cold from a more serious illness, some guides may be helpful.

If a child seems quite sick, if he is lethargic, hard to wake up, uninterested in play or food—he probably has more than a simple cold. Fever is some guide, though again not absolute. High fevers—103 or 104°—seldom go with a simple cold. Symptoms are important too. Earache usually means infection in the ear, not a simple cold; cough, if more than occasional, may indicate infection in throat or chest. Enlarged glands, especially if tender, at the angle of the jaw, suggest a throat infection. These illnesses need a doctor's care. Many are caused, not by viruses, but by bacteria which do respond to drugs, especially the antibiotics. An accurate diagnosis is essential, followed by treatment specific to the particular illness.

A youngster who seems to have a simple cold but who instead of gradually getting better remains sniffly or develops any of the above-mentioned symptoms needs to see a doctor. He may have an illness other than a cold—an allergy or an infection—and he needs treatment from his doctor.

The sad truth is that in this age of miracle medicines when so many truly wonderful things can be done, we are woefully ignorant about either the prevention or the cure of the common cold.

It is not safe for a mother to ignore a cold in her small child. While we have no magic drugs to cure a cold, nevertheless good symptomatic treatment is important in order to prevent a simple cold from becoming a complicated one. In addition, every sniffly nose is not a cold. Colds must be distinguished from more serious diseases, which need specific treatment with drugs from a doctor.

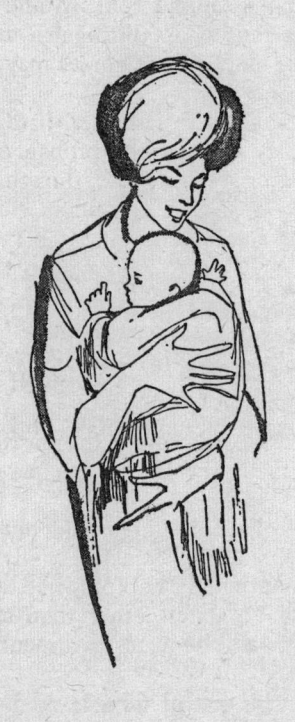

Keep Him Creeping

by Melvin Schrier, O.D., F.A.A.O.

IS your baby son going to Princeton? Have you registered your year-old daughter at Vassar? Most probably many of you have already given much thought to the education of your children. If so, you will be interested in knowing that many professionals in the field of child development believe that the developmental performance of a one year old will seriously affect his future scholastic achievement.

Farfetched? Not really so. It is important to know that a child grows step-by-step—one step at a time, and in a regular and predetermined sequence. It's like building a twenty story building. You must build the first, second and third stories and reinforce them before you can build the fourth floor. If you don't do it properly, the weight of the rest of the sixteen floors will collapse on the poor foundation. So it is with the development of children. It has been shown that children who miss a step in growth, or who don't fully develop each step properly, run into difficulty in school achievement many years later. Perhaps the most important stage to be developed at about the year-old level (and this may normally vary but a few months) is the creeping stage.

This doesn't mean that creeping alone is the key to good school potential but it is at this stage of development that essential coordination and mental processes are also being observed in the child.

According to the Institute of Human Potential in Philadelphia, the creeping stage of development generally takes place between 16 weeks and 60 weeks of life. It is at this stage that the midbrain develops. More meaningful, however, are the following characteristics which develop during this stage. The baby begins to make understandable sounds; he begins to grasp things in his hands; he begins to appreciate details with his vision; he reacts to sounds through his hearing; he begins to understand sensations with his sense of touch. What does all this mean? It indicates that all of his senses are awakening and are beginning to be used. All future sensation—whether it be visual, hearing, touch—will depend on how the child uses his basic abilities at this stage.

More important! What happens if the baby misses this stage? Some, or all, of the senses do not develop properly. In some cases they collapse altogether when the child is placed under stress. The most usual period of stress is at the time when the youngster starts reading at school. It is here that he must use his senses as efficiently and comfortably as possible. If he has built them on a rickety base they will probably collapse at this point—creating the under-achiever, the reading problem, and possibly the school dropout.

How can you avoid the possibility of your child running into this problem in grade school? One answer is to let him creep. Encourage him to creep. Don't rush him into walking.

Play pens are fine when Mommy is busy and can't watch the baby continually. However, his time in the play pen confines the baby so that he cannot creep and offers him easy access to a standing position by the nearness of the rails. This could lead to early walking, without full development of the very important creeping stage.

Creeping can be encouraged by keeping the baby

in the middle of a large room. It should be carpeted preferably so that he will not slip and slide. A baby left in the middle of the floor will eventually do what nature intended him to do—crawl and then creep. If he persists in lying around after the age of eight or nine months, you might entice him by placing his favorite plaything out of his reach. He'll find a way to get to it.

Watch out for grandma! If she's like most grandmas, she will probably want her grandchild to be "way ahead" of other babies on the block. She'll boost him up, she'll walk him around holding him by his hands and be proud when his legs don't collapse under him. Don't argue with her, but when she leaves, put the baby back in the middle of the floor with no visible means of support. He'll walk when he's ready. (After all, no child has crept to the first grade yet!)

Is your child older than the stage we have been discussing? Did he skip the stage wholly or partially? Is he in school having difficulties even though he is of average or better-than average intelligence? Can something be done about it now?

According to the Center for Perceptual Development in New York City and the Institute for Human Potential, children and young adults can be neurologically reorganized (another name for the maturation process we have been discussing). If the problem is diagnosed with special techniques, generally, good results, and sometimes amazing ones, can be attained with a proper training program. Children many grades behind in their achievement level have been brought up to grade level and beyond by retraining very basic development skills. Of course, the younger the child is when his problem is recognized, the easier it usually is to retain him.

However, try to prevent all of this. Encourage your baby to develop at his normal pace. He must be given the opportunity to pass through all the normal stages of development in proper sequence and for a long enough time to create normal patterns of behavior.

If you are concerned about your childs' rate of development, your pediatrician will discuss it with you.

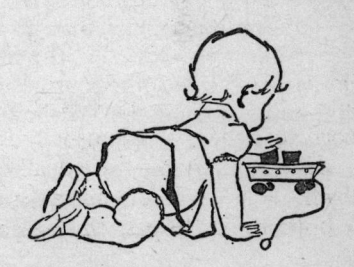

Toilet Training

by Alfred J. Vignec, M.D.

IT cannot be emphasized too strongly that babies are individuals and that they can best be handled as such. This is true of toilet habits as well as of other matters, and a good training program does not fail to take individual differences into consideration.

Almost any mother of two or more children comes to realize very shortly after the birth of the second child that the systems and routines which worked out so well with the first often fail completely, while some patterns and practices which the first baby indignantly rejected are quite acceptable to the new arrival. Perhaps the first baby discarded the night bottle very shortly after coming home from the hospital, and the second clings to it tenaciously. The first could sleep in a noisy, lighted room, while the second demands quiet and semi-darkness. The first was hesitant about accepting solids initially, but the second gobbles them down eagerly from the first day. And so on. Some mothers strive to fit the second baby into the patterns set down by the first, but this is obviously an error. While some routine must be maintained, it should be flexible enough to allow every baby latitude to develop his own personality.

It would be far simpler to write an article on toilet training if all infants were alike in their needs and demands in this particular area. However, any effort to set down absolute rules for time, manner, and method of approaching the training situation invites error, as it will be acceptable to some babies and unacceptable to others. The individual baby must, to some extent, be the guide. Certainly, though, there is general advice to be given for purposes of guidance, especially for the new mother who meets the situation for the first time, or the mother whose second or third child resists training.

It scarcely seems believable now that in our grandmothers' era, toilet training was started at 3 or 4 months of age. The infant was held over a tiny potty until his bowel movement was accomplished, and he was often fully trained to bowel control within a few months. It is quite true that this is possible, but it is frowned upon. Many grandparents insist that no severe damage was done by such early training methods, but psychologists and physicians feel strongly that an undue strain was imposed on the nervous system of the young infant by the effort to train him to control his bowel and bladder functions in any way at all.

The point in a good program, then, is the matter of age. Toilet training should not be begun until the baby is able to sit freely without support of any kind. In most infants this is accomplished by about ten months—however, some sit earlier, some later. When toilet training is begun at this time, the mother must remember that she and she alone is responsible for the routine, since the infant does not understand what it is all about. Only the baby with very regular bowel patterns is ready for training at this period. If the infant has his movements directly after meals, for example, the mother may put him on the infant toilet seat or potty chair and wait for a short period of time to see whether he reacts. No force or even undue coaxing should be used. He cannot really be taught to control himself as yet. His understanding has not developed enough. Success depends on what we call a "conditioned response", or what may be more simply described as a "habit." He will not ask to go, even if he is an early talker and has mastered several simple words. If he soils, it is either due to an error in the mother's judgment or to some inner disruption of his usual routine. NEVER can the young baby be held responsible.

It is often preferable to wait with training until the baby stands and walks freely. The reason for this is primarily that at this period bowel patterns may change and since the infant is still not old enough to ask, the whole procedure may have to be started over. Even now the training program still rests entirely with the mother. It is she who must notice when the baby has to go to the bathroom. The child who is fully trained at a relatively young age may suddenly begin to soil or wet again. This lapse is usually only temporary and with a little patience, soon disappears.

In some cases it is advisable to postpone training entirely until the baby has some idea of what it is all about. This is best for the baby who is less regular in his habits or reacts with marked reluctance or confusion when earlier training is attempted. The fifteen month old is very rarely able to let his mother know he wants to go to the bathroom ahead of time, but frequently he will let her know AFTER his pants are already wet. While this seems to be of little use, it does indicate that he himself is beginning to become aware of his messiness and is ready to have something done about it. It shows, too, that he is able to cooperate to some extent in the training program—it is no longer only a "conditioned response" or habit pattern.

In deciding when to institute training, the mother should be guided by the bowel patterns and abilities of her baby, not in any degree by a desire to avoid diaper mess. Toilet training is too important a part of the child's personality formation to be influenced by the mother's urge to have him out of diapers. Occasionally a mother waits until the child can ask before training at all. If the reason for this is genuinely the child's own welfare, it may work out satisfactorily, but too often very late training is caused by the mother's reluctance to handle the training situation—in this case it may result in a very trying period when the child is socially unacceptable, embarrassed, and even unhappy. A child who is different from others of his own age often feels inferior and grows shy or resentful. Except in unusual cases, training should be started between the tenth and sixteenth months of age.

What is the best method? Actually, both toilet seat and potty chair are satisfactory. The seat is perhaps less troublesome and is acceptable if the adult toilet to which it is attached can be kept sanitary since the baby will, of course, rest his hands on the adult seat quite frequently. The potty chair, if sturdily built, allows the mother more freedom of movement, as she may supervise the child without having to stay in the bathroom. Many babies resent both seat and chair, initially. Others will not soil or wet when their diapers are off, as they do not feel this to be the "correct" thing to do. These resistances can be overcome by patience. If the child resists he should not be forced. Training should be stopped for a few days or weeks then tried again. At all costs, the mother should avoid making a contest of it.

It is not wise to leave the baby on the potty or seat for more than 10-20 minutes at a time. Also, if at all possible, toys, cookies, lollypops, etc. should be avoided while the child is on the potty in order to prevent the habit of dawdling there and not performing unless he has what he wants at the moment. The sooner he finishes and is free to leave, the better. Using the potty chair for other purposes entirely (such as play or feeding when it is not in use as a potty), is also unwise, as the baby should come to think of it as a toilet only. His habits will be better defined and more efficient if this can be carried out.

Toilet training should be made a natural part of the

day's routine. The mother should not be too eager, nor too disappointed at failure. Accidents for the entire first year of training should be anticipated. Bowel training is accomplished first, generally, and bowel "accidents" are far less frequent than wetting. Bladder training is more difficult and is very rarely accomplished before the baby can ask. Even then he is not usually a good judge of his own abilities, and will often play too long, ask too late, or, when out, forget to ask until he is miles from a toilet. The trained child is often badly upset by an unexpected "accident" and should be comforted and reassured rather than scolded. In fact, from start to finish of the toilet training program, the mother should always praise the baby generously for succeeding but should not blame him for his failures. Such blame tends to make him timid, tense, or even angry. The timid or tense child will often wet when he tries not to; the angry child can retain even his bowel movements and not go to the bathroom at all for quite a while, or can wet and soil at will to "spite" the mother. This seems like quite a nasty bit of calculating, but the child often acts instinctively and does not even realize what he is doing.

It is always well to remember that infants and children (like most adults) do not like force and will tend to resist it in one way or another. Once the child feels that the mother is trying to force him and he is trying to outwit her, a contest has been started and often the parents find themselves up against quite a problem, as children can think of many conscious and unconscious weapons for frustrating and defeating adults. The best thing to do from the start is win the child's cooperation. If he wants to please you, he will help you to teach him, whatever the training program may be.

At all ages, the mother should try to keep the child's bowels regular with proper amounts of fruit, etc. If he is well, it helps in his training.

TOILET TRAINING

Roughly, his abilities run as follows, dependent always on his own patterns of walking and talking:

10 months—can sit on potty or seat, if placed
15 months—can indicate wet diapers. May be trained. Will not ask.
21 months—asks
24 months—dry if taken up at night (Still may have accidents)

If the child over three who was fully trained, reverts to patterns of bedwetting it is called "enuresis." This is usually the result of emotional upset.

Whenever possible, the same person should teach the baby his toilet habits. The less emphasis placed on accidents and the more praise for accomplishing his purpose, the more rapidly he will be trained. He should not be punished. The child's attention should be attracted to his wetting of the floor or his pants while he is being bladder trained and he should realize this is not what is expected, but he should not be shamed. When dry pants are put on him the dryness should be emphasized ("There, now you're dry again."), so that he realizes wet pants are not pleasant. If the child asks and no attention is paid him, it is the mother's fault if he wets.

Some children are trained rapidly and easily, others find it more difficult. Problems which arise can usually be dealt with without too much trouble. The mother, above all, should strive to remain calm in this as well as other situations, as the baby is aways aware of the mother's frustration. If the mother despairs of ever being able to train him, after a series of delays for one reason or another, the baby too loses confidence and the program of training may distintegrate entirely for a while. If, on the other hand, the mother accepts failures cheerfully, the baby draws confidence from her, and the failures diminish.

It is well always to remember that the baby wants to

conform, to win approval and to be loved. A baby who seems to be setting out to rebel, to frustrate and defeat his parents is doing so only because he does not feel able to please.

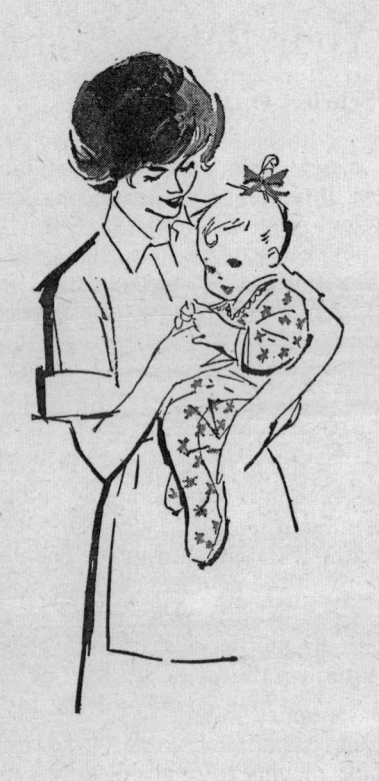

Your Baby's Sight

by Melvin Schrier, O.D., F.A.A.O.

WITH a new baby, you are concerned with all manner of unaccustomed problems. But you don't want to overlook your role in helping baby use his eyes properly as he grows. When a baby is born, he is born with the ability to look, but in order to see, he must learn many things and start to store up all the memories that he will have for a lifetime. Because vision is a learned process, all the help we can give him will show dividends later in life.

The first reaction a baby's eyes will have is to light. He will start to notice the difference between light and shadow. It's a good idea to place one of those nice new lamps in the baby's room. No, not for reading yet, but it will hold a 15-watt bulb that can be left on in the room, so that the baby will have this lighted area to look at whenever he wakes up. And every once in a while, change his position in the crib, and change the position of the crib, so that he can develop both sides of his new body.

A special mobile should hang over Junior's crib. After lights and shadows become "baby-stuff," he will have something moving to catch his eyes.

You know all those rattles that were tied to the presents you got? Well, these novelties are going to help your infant, too. How? Baby learns to see from himself on out. In other words, his world starts at his hands and expands to the room, to the house, and the world beyond.

The rattle will give him a chance to feel and see at the same time. The bright color and the noise will help him orient his senses—touch, hearing, seeing. In order to grow properly, the coordination of his eyes and hands and body should become smooth and easy. The little rattle will be a start.

By the time he is four months old, the rattle becomes a nice, smooth object to put in his mouth. This is a very important experience in his attempts to coordinate all his senses. Babies like to grasp small blocks of wood or plastic and bang them together. (Now you'll have to help him, but he'll do it alone when he's about 10 months old.) The noise will make his eyes turn towards his hands, another way of encouraging hand-eye coordination. The small cubes that you get for Junior at this time will be a "long term investment." All through his growing months and years he'll find many ways to use them in play.

If your baby develops about the same as other four-month old babies, he should be about ready to help you hold his bottle during feeding time. Of course, you'll have to place his hands in the proper position. This will help him to know where his hands are in relation to his mouth, with some assistance from his eyes.

Because a five-month old is primarily concerned with things close to his body, now will be a good time to move his mobile towards him. His new explorations will include some pulling, releasing and even breaking of his toys. Don't brag too much about the strong man; just make sure you have provided him with safe, unbreakable playthings. In addition to having his hands grasp, help him use his legs by teaching him to kick at the mobile.

When his half-anniversary rolls around, he should start to recognize differences between Uncle Gene and Uncle Richard. This would be a good time to introduce him to some young playmates. He will like to watch them move around, move towards him and away from him, starting his awareness of size and distance differences.

This is also the time he may start to creep. It's also time for a ball. Get him a large, colorful ball to attract his attention while he's crawling around in his play pen. The process of reaching for it will help in his muscular development. Take advantage of this stage—in a little while you'll have to chase him all over the house!

In another month or so, that ball of string you've been saving is going to come in handy. Attach a long string to all his toys. This is the stage when things get thrown from the high chair. The string will save your back, but it's important to let Junior play his "game" to the limit. He wants to watch a toy drop, and to hear the noise it makes. He doesn't know it, but he is really learning what "down" is.

When baby's first birthday rolls around, grandma, grandpa and all the family will be straining to understand the sounds that he makes all day long. About this time, too, you are going to find him in all corners of the house. This is his way of expanding his space world by exploring as far as he can.

It's not usually necessary to take the baby to have his eyes checked professionally, but it is important to watch his eyes all through his development to see if everything is progressing well. You are certainly not going to worry if Junior is a few weeks or so behind the so-called "normals," and you are not going to boast—too much—if he's two weeks ahead of his cousin. But, if something looks really wrong, it's a good idea to thoroughly check by the time he is seven or eight months old.

Normally, you'll wait until he's four, or at the latest, five years old to get his first vision examination. But it's your job to start him properly now!

Your Child's Feet

by Morton H. Walker, D.S.C.

YOUR child's feet are the foundation on which his whole body will grow strong and straight. If your child is average, he will be born with strong feet 80% of the time. He is able to keep them that way, but only with your help.

Sometimes a baby's foot problem is overlooked in the general physical examination. Also, it may be disregarded when you take him to buy a pair of shoes. Do you realize that shoes are the one article of clothing that can cripple your child and cause him to have a foot problem for life? You must buy shoes with the utmost care and have them fitted carefully, just as you would glasses or a hearing aid.

Your child may suffer from one of the common foot problems like pigeon toeing, knocked knees, bow legs, painful heels, flat feet or toe walking. These are all manifested by various symptoms that your baby plainly shows to you. He may dislike walking or running, or he may take off his shoes frequently. He may wake up at night crying from pain in his feet or legs. He may walk with an unusual gait, or fall down frequently, or just stumble over his own feet. He may not rise easily from the floor. If any of these physical problems show themselves, then it is possible your child is suffering from improper foot hygiene, the wrong kind of shoes, or a congenital foot fault.

Parents and teachers can catch these symptoms early and aid the youngster to grow up on sound feet. If you see your child walk with a kind of "Charlie Chaplin gait" complicated by knocked knees, then look at his heel tendons from behind and you might see that they are slightly bowed inward. This is a symptom of pronation or weak feet. It is treatable and correctable by a foot specialist.

In pigeon toeing, bow legs are usually a complication. Then the foot doctor uses a Denis Brown Bar with shoes attached. The child sleeps with this bar on at night and the end result is usually straight legs and corrected feet.

Toe walking may be no serious problem or it could arise from strain or apophysitis. If it continues, flat feet and a short heel tendon could develop. It should be investigated.

One thing to remember is never put your child in his brother's or sister's worn, hand-me-down shoes. The worn shoe has already taken on the shape of the other child's feet. It will cause Junior to walk in an unusual pattern so that he may bring on a foot problem that wasn't there before.

Gifts of baby booties and tiny sleeper socks may be welcomed by you, but you have to make sure that they have plenty of room to spare for those wiggly toes to grow. The baby's feet grow so fast that you must check once a week to make sure there is enough room.

Baby's first real shoes are of the pre-walker type. This is a boot with a flexible sole and a soft upper leather. These shoes are mainly for crawling rather than walking.

High shoes are necessary for first walkers. The feet of babies are small, sensitive and not developed. They need the protection around the ankles that high shoes give. Also, the baby cannot take his shoes off as most of them try to do. Low shoes tend to slip off easily from the baby's feet. The first walker is a hard sole of leather or composition that is just flexible enough for balance.

The fitting of children's shoes is a most important function. It should be done with integrity and sincere interest. In fitting children's shoes, the fit is only as dependable as the shoe fitter. It is imperative that you find a shoe store with high standards, trained personnel and a reputation for honesty.

A child's shoes should be checked every three months to make sure he has not outgrown them before he has outworn them. If there is growth room, a reputable shoe store will not try to sell you a pair of shoes just to put money in the cash register.

At different ages, shoe sizes change in proportion to the speed of growth of the whole child. On the average, children ages one to six change sizes in four to eight weeks; ages six to ten change sizes in eight to twelve weeks; ages ten to twelve change sizes in twelve to sixteen weeks; age twelve to fifteen change sizes in sixteen to twenty weeks.

Children's shoe sections of department stores and special children's shoe stores keep a file system recording the date of their small customer's last visit and shoe sizes purchased. A service making use of this card system to remind you of your child's last visit, indicates that the store has a sincere interest and will give you the attention you need for proper shoe fitting.

Shoe sizes vary from one brand to the next, mainly because the factory uses different shapes of lasts. So fit shoes by feel rather than by numbers. It is important to have plenty of length and width.

Some shoe fitters may mean well when they suggest a correction for a minor foot disorder. But your foot doctor is the only person who can prescribe or diagnose for a foot problem. The shoe salesman who recommends incorporation of a scaphoid pad or an outside sole wedge is practicing podiatry without a license. He may be doing it as much for the extra money it brings him as for the foot correction. He is not trained for this practice, and he is committing a crime against you, your child and society.

Barefoot walking is good. It promotes strong healthy feet when bare-footedness is restricted to grass, sand, soft earth or carpeted floors. Barefoot romping on concrete, hardwood floors, asphalt tile or rocks is definitely to be discouraged. Walking barefoot on these hard, flat unyielding surfaces only leads to foot strain and future foot problems.

If your child has a foot problem, the foot doctor will probably not allow him to wear sneakers because they give only partial support to the feet and are not made to hold corrections. Therefore, the writer feels that healthy feet can wear sneakers and weak feet should not wear them because they do nothing to enhance correction.

A child's arch forms at about age two and a half years. That is when his ankle, foot and leg have developed more, and he is able to wear low cut shoes or oxfords. His stockings, too, should have sufficient room for growth and stretching of the toes, but not so much room that they gather and bunch-up under the toes. There are proper foot exercises that can be made use of as a game to strengthen the toes, arches and muscles of children with weak feet. If you mention to your podiatrist that you are interested in some exercises he will recommend the following:

1. The child should stand on a book or over the edge of a step and bend the toes down and up as far as possible.
2. He should walk around the room for five minutes on the outer edges of his feet.
3. He should grasp marbles with the toes and hold them contracted and walk around the room on his heels.
4. He should rise up on his tiptoes and slowly lower himself down.

5. He should stand near a wall with his arms outstretched so that when he falls forward stiff-legged his elbows will bend and support him on the wall. He should keep his heels flat so that he puts a stretch on his calf muscles.
6. He should attempt to kick himself with his heels. This will help his thigh muscles.
7. He should sit in the chair and roll his foot arches on a Coca Cola bottle.

The writer recommends that children's shoes not be repaired. It is more economical that shoes be repaired, but when a shoemaker, even a skilled one, repairs a shoe, he almost invariably makes it smaller. It is far better to invest the repair money in new shoes to make sure the shoe size is correct at all times.

There are certain rules for parents to remember when supervising your child's foot health:

1. Periodic foot check-ups are every bit as important to a child's health as periodic physical or dental check-ups.
2. Never let your child wear hand-me-down shoes.
3. Let him walk barefoot only on soft surfaces.
4. Let him wear sneakers if he has healthy feet; shoes if he does not.
5. Make sure socks are long enough.
6. Watch for any unusual sign or symptoms of foot and leg fatigue.
7. If there is any suspicion that there is a leg or foot problem, take your child to a foot specialist.
8. Find a reputable shoe fitter and stay with him.

Children between ages two to eight take about 30,000 steps a day. With all this walking, running and jumping, it is a wonder that they don't suffer from foot problems more often. When foot trouble does arise, more than 70% of it can be corrected immediately, especially if it is recognized early. The diagnosis and correction of a foot problem is in the province of the podiatrist, the pediatrician and the orthopedic surgeon. You must not make your own diagnosis or depend on the unskilled eye of the shoe fitter to determine whether a child has or has not a foot problem. If a child is to be helped early in his formative years, it is imperative that you, the parent, seek the proper professional guidance. Remember—your children's feet are in your hands.

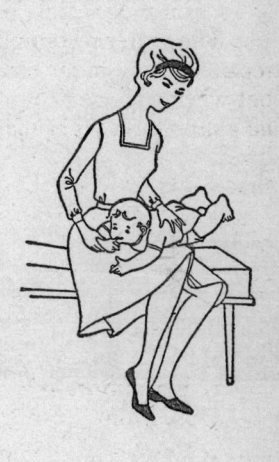

Immunization Chart

by **Frank Howard Richardson, M.D.**

WE are living in an age of medical miracles—and how many of us realize how truly miraculous this age is? It is not many years ago that parents saw epidemics of contagious diseases attacking whole communities. Diphtheria did untold harm in our grandparent's day—in our own time, polio was a dreaded killer.

The biggest problem parents face today is to remember what immunizations are necessary—for their babies and young children—and to keep an accurate record of the dates when immunizations or booster shots should be given. Even though your doctor or pediatrician will himself have such a record, your own timetable will be important as your child grows, and finally attends school.

Elsewhere in this book you will find a Health Record which will help you keep your Immunization Timetable accurately. The following schedule of immunizations will safely see your baby through infancy and the toddler years.

At three months: First quadruple vaccination against diphtheria, tetanus, whooping cough and polio.

At four months: A second quadruple vaccination against the same four diseases.

At five months: A third quadruple vaccination.

At ten months: Measles vaccination.

At one year: Smallpox vaccination and tuberculin test.
Between 14 & 18 months: Fourth quadruple vaccination.
At two years: A tuberculin test.
At four years: Another quadruple vaccination and a tuberculin test.

There may be occasions when your own physician may want to change this timetable. Defer to his decisions, of course, since he knows your child.

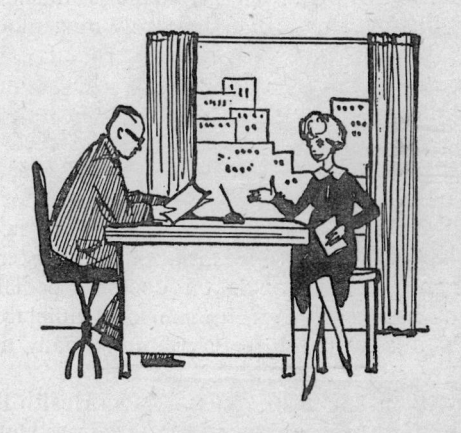

SECTION IV

Feeding and Nutrition

Modern Feeding Practices

by Elizabeth D. Munves, Ph.D.

A mother's first association with her new baby is often at feeding time. Whether this is her first baby or her fifth, a mother soon realizes that each baby is an individual with his own set of built-in ideas about his food. It is amazing that these characteristics show at such an early age: some babies are so hungry they are miserable, others suck steadily and rather slowly, while another may be satisfied with small amounts more frequently. By the time most mothers leave the hospital, they have begun to know their baby's eating pattern. The care and feeding of each new baby needs to be fitted into the existing routine of the household. Unless this is done smoothly, feeding problems can arise later on.

Don't forget that a baby at birth is nine months old, as feeding actually begins at conception. In addition, the general health picture of the mother before conception greatly influences the course of a successful pregnancy. Many processes, such as the formation of teeth, are dependent upon good nutritional supplies during pregnancy. So, as one authority stated, the life cycle (and the nutrition cycle) is never broken.

Each mother must decide for herself whether she is going to breast feed her baby or to feed it by bottle. A new mother can list many advantages of breast feeding but a few stand out as being more important. A mother is sure that it is safe and there is no danger of contamination. She knows that she can provide the necessary nutrients in the proper amount. Also, she is certain to devote precious time to her baby.

Although many clinicians will state that breast feeding is the "best" way to feed a newborn, they are quick to add that they have no evidence to support the statement today other than that it should be best because it is the food designed for the human baby, just as the breast milk of other species is the accepted food for its young. Thus the many factors that may be responsible for the superior value of breast milk are not fully defined.

A majority of mothers choose to feed their babies by formula. This is due, in part, to the simplicity and safety of artificial feeding. In addition, babies who have been bottle fed on properly constructed formulas thrive and perform equally as well as infants receiving human milk. The human infant receives its immunity from the mother before birth by way of the placenta. Thus, a formerly held belief concerning the unique advantage of breast feeding has been disproved.

Breast milk isn't "naturally" adequate. Some mothers have the mistaken notion that regardless of diet, as long as they are able to produce milk, it will be "all right." Nutritionally adequate milk depends largely upon the diet and health of the mother. The nursing mother should include the following in her menu each day to be sure her mik contains enough protein, vitamins, minerals, and calories:

```
milk .................................. 1½ quarts
citrus fruit or tomato ........ 2 servings
lean meat, fish, poultry ...... 2 servings of
                                approximately 4 ounces
egg ........................................... 1
leafy, green vegetable ........ at least one serving
```

plus other foods such as breads, other fruits and vegetables, and the "extra" foods to provide an adequate number of calories.

Nutrition-wise the two milks compare favorably. Newer techniques in food processing have reduced the curd tension in cow's milk so that the protein becomes readily available. Formerly it was held that the protein in human milk was biologically superior to that in cow's milk formulas. In constructing the formula, the fat and carbohydrate content approximate that of human milk. Both breast milk and cow's milk contain adequate amounts of calcium, vitamin A, riboflavin, and niacin.

However, there is some variation in nutritive value. Breast milk is sufficiently rich in ascorbic acid provided the mother includes enough vitamin C in her diet (see the foods listed). But ascorbic acid in the form of citrus fruits is usually added to the diet of both bottle-fed and breast-fed infants during the first month of life. Although the iron found in human milk is more readily absorbed than that of cow's milk, neither provides sufficient amounts. It has long been recognized that the infant is born with a store of iron adequate for the first three or four months of life. The thiamine content of both types of milk is low. The addition of cereal and then egg yolk to the infant's diet will provide these needed nutrients, iron and thiamine, in sufficient time. Vitamin D is given within the first month of life, whether the baby is fed by breast or bottle.

Many physicians believe that there is a psychological advantage to both the mother and the child in breast feeding. However, others feel that this same feeling can be experienced as a mother bottle feeds her baby if she holds him in the same manner. It must be emphasized that the temptation to prop the bottle with a pillow or to use the "bottle holders" while so-called necessary household duties are performed should be resisted. One of the dividends about bottle fed babies is that fathers can "get into the act." They can have the fun of sharing some of the care of the baby and establish a warm relationship during an infant's early life.

In recent years emphasis has been placed on the psychological as well as the nutritional aspects of feeding. The "demand" feeding, or, to use the preferred term, "self-regulating" feeding illustrates this point of view. Bakwin enumerated three aspects of self-regulation in feeding the infant: (1) the interval between feedings (2) the amount of food, and (3) the type of food.

Thus the infant determines whether he shall have a feeding at regular intervals, such as every four hours, or if he shall eat at a three hour interval at one time and five or six hour interval at another. He sets his own pattern in regard to giving up feedings at night. This approach is often difficult for the young mother who feels more secure in waking the baby for his "ten o'clock bottle."

The baby, too, determines the amount of food he will take. This may vary considerably from feeding to feeding. The mother who nurses can accept this idea more readily as she is unaware of the exact number of ounces that baby has taken. No amount of urging seems to be able to force a full, contented baby to drink additional milk. Usually the amount of food a baby desires will vary from feeding to feeding, yet be relatively consistent from day to day. The activity of the baby, such as waving his hands and legs, will often influence the amount of each feeding.

As he grows older and foods are introduced, a baby will indicate a decided preference for one food over another. Sometimes he is adamant about the order in which he eats his food. A baby of eight weeks can clearly tell his mother that he wants to drink a few ounces of milk before he readily accepts cereal. Another infant will prefer cereal first. Expressed likes and dislikes concerning vegetables, fruits, cereals, etc. are not necessarily permanent at this age.

"No fuss—no bother" might well be the theme of the mother who bottle feeds her infant today. Many new products help to make life easier. Prepared formulas have been on the market for many years, yet there is now a greater variety for the physician to select from. Others are packaged in disposable bottles, ready to unwrap and safely hand to the baby without warming them.

Recently physicians have introduced many innovations in the feeding of infants. While terminal sterilization, a greatly simplified way of sterilizing the bottle, nipple and formula simultaneously, has been practiced for some time, some are suggesting that the formula be made without sterilization. All equipment must still be scrupulously clean, but the formula is made with tap water and then fed to the baby. Many babies are given regular milk soon after they leave the hospital, thus bypassing the formula stage. An even greater change is the evidence that babies seem to get along just as well on cold formulas as warmed ones! While each physician decides what is best for those babies in his care, these changes in infant feeding are gaining wider acceptance.

When are solid foods introduced in the infant's diet? You will find a different pattern practiced by each clinician . . . and these are probably varied from baby to baby. One doctor reports on an early feeding schedule he has supervised with many hundreds of babies. He introduces cereals at two or three days, quickly adds other solid foods, such as meat, vegetables, fruit. At approximately 17 days the babies are on three meals a day, and by 9 weeks an infant might be enjoying a full breakfast of bacon and eggs. Others point out that the sucking motion is important to the infant's psychological development and that it takes several weeks before the baby is able to transfer food from the front of his mouth to the back without choking.

Not only is there wide difference in opinion about when foods are introduced in the infant's diet, but there is no general agreement concerning the order in which foods are added. All usually recommend orange juice followed by cereal as good starter foods. But whether fruits, vegetables or meats are introduced next depends upon the opinion of the individual doctor.

When solids are added to the infant's diet, the mother has a wealth of products from which to choose; egg yolk, an increasing variety of meats, cereals fortified with vitamins, minerals, and protein, and many combinations of foods. Again, an important commodity, time, has been saved for the busy mother.

Scientific advances have dictated the trends in infant feeding. Our babies today are stronger, better developed, and healthier than those of former days. It is hoped that the changing trends in infant feeding have contributed, in part, to this development.

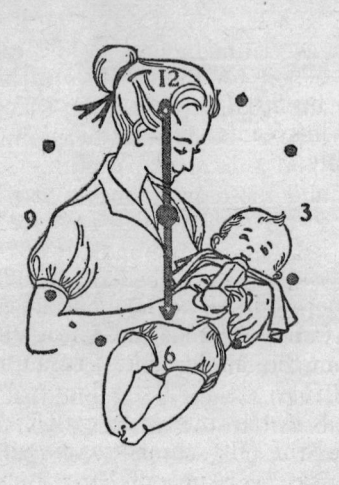

Introducing New Foods

by Elizabeth D. Munves, Ph.D.

MOTHERS enjoy feeding their children. Yet questions about foods seem to be a major concern. Even an experienced mother has uneasy moments when she thinks of caring for her new baby. She may be able to distinguish the infant's hunger cry from his other demands, she may know such things as how to hold a new baby, the best temperature for milk and so on, but each baby is an individual. A mother needs to learn about him—his likes and dislikes (yes, they seem to be there at birth!), his rate of eating, his sleep pattern, and many other things. Above all, the care and feeding of each new baby has to be fitted into the existing routine of the household. Thus feeding problems can arise unless this is done smoothly.

Why is infant feeding so important during the first year? True, you are providing necessary nutrients for this period of rapid growth. But you also need to acquaint your baby with variations in the taste, texture and temperature of foods, so that, at the end of his first year, he will accept a variety of foods and is ready to eat most of the foods from the family table. One authority pointed out that—"Babies are usually willing to try out many different foods in the six months period following weaning, but after this, the number approved gradually declines, and picks up again only after a child gets to be six or seven."

A child's attitude toward food can be strongly influenced by the way he is fed during his first year of life. Forget about what the "baby down the block" is eating! How, when, and what your baby is fed is determined by him, your doctor and you. Too often, well-meaning friends and relatives succeed in promoting a sense of competition among mothers regarding food. Since each child develops physically at his own rate of speed, introducing foods must be related to this.

Milk is your baby's first food. Like other young animals, he is born with rooting, suckling and swallowing reflexes, he quickly accepts milk. During early weeks, the timing and amount appear to be erratic. A baby may vigorously take a large feeding one time and a smaller amount another time. There seems no way of predicting how much each child will drink.

Babies usually swallow air as they suck. So, whether he is breast or bottle fed be sure to "burp" him after each ounce. This will remove air bubbles that can cause distressing pain.

The nutrients supplied by milk are protein, varying amounts of the B vitamins and minerals. It is very low in vitamin C. Thus, the first food added to this milk diet is usually the juice of a citrus fruit. Any of the citrus group may be used. Tomato juice also contains vitamin C, though only about a quarter as much as orange juice. Strained diluted juice is offered at first, and gradually the baby is able to have full strength two-three ounce feedings.

A source of vitamin D is also added during the first few weeks of life. This may be in the form of drops. Or, your doctor may decide that fortified milk (if that is what you are using) may supply enough vitamin D.

There is no set time table when "solid" foods are introduced. It can vary in age from two weeks to six months. You are asking your baby to learn many new things: to take food from a spoon, to carry food from the front of his mouth, and to swallow a "lump", quite different from the fluid milk. So don't expect him to take to it—as the famous duck to water!

Cereal is often the first solid food offered. You may either use one prepared for your whole family or one of the instant baby cereals. If cooked at home, select one that is highly refined and cook it thoroughly. Thin the cereal with a little of the baby's formula. At first it should be so thin that it can run off the end of a spoon. If you offer a little cereal on the end of a spoon he may suck it off. Too, the tongue acting as a guardian may at first push out anything just inside the baby's lips. So, don't be alarmed if he refuses your first attempts at giving solid food.

In time, the amount and kinds of cereals increase. Again, each baby will let you know his favorite cereals and the size portion he desires. Besides calories, cereals contribute small amounts of the B vitamins and iron to the diet.

When the baby is readily accepting cereal, fruit may be the next offering. Again, you may use fruits from the family table or buy the ready-prepared baby fruits. If you prepare them yourself, be sure they are thoroughly cooked and strained. Fruits contain so much natural sweetness that you needn't add sugar.

Most babies love fruits. Applesauce or a mashed ripe banana (select a dark skin) are a popular first choice. Offer this after cereal and milk or alternate tastes of familiar foods with unfamiliar ones. Don't mix them all together—for then your baby won't learn to develop different tastes.

Vegetables are introduced at a meal when neither cereal nor fruit are offered. Most babies prefer mild to strong flavors. A word of caution: vegetables spoil quickly. Unless your baby can finish a new jar, never feed him from the jar itself. Instead, warm a small amount in a custard cup and keep the unused portion refrigerated.

Soon your baby will be eating from two to three tablespoons of his favorite vegetables each day. Both vegetables and fruits, depending upon the food itself, supply varying amounts of vitamins, minerals and calories.

Babies are born with a few month's store of iron. So when egg yolk is added to the diet at three to five months, it supplies this nutrient. It also provides protein and vitamins. A cooked egg yolk can be given in many ways: in cereal, alone, or as a custard. You may use the canned yolk or the fresh. If the latter, cook it thoroughly. Many babies are allergic to egg white, so your doctor may withhold this until your baby is from nine to twelve months.

The time that meats are added to a baby's diet varies according to your doctor's orders. Jars of strained meats, scraped beef, or finely mashed meats add variety, flavor and texture to menus. Crisp bacon adds little of the nutrients found in meats (protein, minerals, and vitamins), but most babies like its flavor.

During the second six months of the baby's first year gradually change the finely pureed foods to coarsely chopped ones. The baby needs to begin to chew, even if he hasn't teeth. Dry bread, zwieback, big pretzel sticks and the like also encourage the chewing reflex. Soft breads should be avoided until he has learned to chew well.

Contrary to popular notion, a baby doesn't need sweets. He does need calories (as well as other nutrients) so by the end of the first year he can begin having simple desserts, like custards and puddings, that have little sugar to give him additional calories.

Remember, not only are you providing nutrients, but you are developing attitudes toward food that will remain with your baby throughout life.

A Commonsense Feeding Program

by **Walter W. Sackett, Jr., M.D.**

BREAST *Feeding*. Aside from convenience, your milk is better for your baby than cow's milk. It's also better for your baby than the milk from another mother, (a wet nurse) because of the natural affinity of each baby to its mother. In short, your milk is tailor-made for your baby. Authorities on infant nutrition agree that mother's milk carries with it an immunity against certain diseases, extending the natural immunity inherited from the mother at birth, and that this factor is credited with the lower incidence of illness among breast-fed babies.

Even when a mother has decided to feed by bottle, I recommend that she breast-feed her baby at least for the first few days or weeks. This recommendation is made in her interest as well as the baby's; the suckling action on the breasts helps the uterus to contract and return to its normal position—probably by exciting hormones secreted by the pituitary glands—just as nature intended. Also, a better psychological relationship develops between mother and baby in a breast-feeding schedule; the two will develop a greater spirit of togetherness, and the mother will have fewer unexplained aches and pains if a period of twenty or thirty minutes is spent at each feeding time in the privacy of nursing. And too, it is reported that breast cancer occurs less frequently among mothers who nurse their babies.

Combination Breast and Bottle. It frequently happens that a mother who is breast-feeding her baby must be absent from home for a few hours. Mothers who return to work can nurse their babies each morning and evening, preparing a bottle feeding for the noon meal. Similarly a mother who wants to attend a sorority luncheon can leave a bottle with the baby-sitter. It may make you feel more comfortable, and give you better peace of mind if you empty your breast by hand or with a breast pump at about the time of the scheduled feeding which is not given. It may also make you feel more at ease if you prepare baby for the new kind of milk by giving him a bottle feeding a day or two before your expected absence, just to see how he accepts it. This is really necessary; he'll drink from the bottle if he's hungry enough, and if he's not he can wait until you get home again. Occasionally a baby may rebel at breast feeding once he has experienced bottle feeding, since the bottle requires much less effort on his part, but this is not worth worrying over.

Weaning. The changeover from breast or bottle to cup usually can be accomplished between the ages of eight months and a year. It can be done even earlier if water is offered in a cup at three and a half to five months of age, as soon as baby can hold his head up. The result will seem sloppy at first, because baby isn't skilled at taking liquids except by sucking, and his attempt to suck at the cup's edge will be somewhat in the nature of a drool. But have patience! The little tyke will catch on quite quickly is you give him half a chance. In a short time he'll prefer his newfound method of drinking liquids to the old one, and he'll eagerly learn to hold the cup himself. He'll have accidents, of course, but he'll be learning. To avoid getting your floors wet, it's a good idea to let baby have his first practice sessions at drinking from a cup while he's in the bathtub, where a little spilled water won't hurt a thing. Some babies, to be sure, show no interest in the cup until nine or ten months of age. This isn't anything worth worrying over; it merely proves the old adage that we are not all alike.

Milk given from a cup should be at room temperature and have the smallest possible fat content, causing me to prefer the nonfat dry milk, reconstituted with water. For practice sessions between meals, water should be offered rather than milk, in keeping with the standing rule that only water should be allowed between the regularly scheduled meals.

Adaptation, Right from the Start. Babies born in hospitals, as almost all of them are nowadays, start off on a feeding schedule that is established as much for the convenience of hospital personnel as for the baby's welfare. Some hospitals offer feedings at four-hour intervals, usually selecting the hours of 2:00, 6:00, and 10:00 A.M.; and 2:00, 6:00, and 10:00 P.M. The hour of birth is not taken into consideration.

In my hospital practice, I have found that four feedings a day are adequate, and they are given at the hours of 6:00, 12:00—6:00, 12:00, again because these are the most workable ones in keeping with hospital routine. At these times we offer the baby bottle or breast, according to the mother's wishes and considerations outlined here. If the bottle is used, we use the regular hospital formula. If indicated for any reason, and this seldom occurs, we supplement the breat feeding with a bottle. If the mother is particularly intent on nursing, we urge her not to give the supplementary bottle and to give ample water (but only once!) between meals. This with the solid foods that we add to his diet, gives the baby all the substance he needs to grow on.

At 2 to 3 Days, Cereal. You'll probably find it convenient to give cereal at 6:00 A.M. and 6:00 P.M. in order to fit the baby into the family schedule most efficiently. It should be prepared with only enough formula to achieve the semisolid consistency of putty. There are several kinds of already cooked starter cereal for babies available, and I recommend barley, rice or oatmeal for the initial meals.

Cereal should be given at the beginning of the feeding before milk. Use a moderate amount on the tip of the spoon so that you're giving only about a quarter-teaspoonful at first. You will quickly discover how best to maneuver the food into his mouth. It is the usual thing for him to take it into his mouth, move it around in an exploratory manner, and gradually swallow it; rarely will he resist. Three or four of these quarter-teaspoon "servings" will suffice for the first cereal feeding. Unless there is some sign of intolerance by next day, you can increase the quantity to as much as he will take.

At 10 Days—strained vegetables are added to the noon meal. There are several brands of prepared baby food offered in cans and jars. Carrots, peas, string beans, or squash are good choices for the first vegetable feeding, and the preparation of the commercial baby foods is simple. While I urge that foods should be served at room temperature, they may be heated, either by placing the jar or can in boiling water or by removing the contents and heating them in a small saucepan. I am inclined to favor the in-the-jar method because it eliminates the additional utensil which can possibly carry germs and in any case must be cleaned afterward.

At 14 Days, Strained Meats are offered either at noon, along with the vegetables, or at 6:00 P.M. with the cereal feeding. There is something different or new about meat, either in texture or taste, that sometimes prompts an infant to push meat from his mouth with his tongue. An easy solution to this is to feed him in layers—that is, to offer first the meat and then quickly follow it with a small bit of some previously accepted vegetable. As a matter of fact, this is how most of us enjoy our food, too—a bit of meat and then one of vegetable. Possibly newer meat preparations, tastier and of a finer consistency, will solve this minor problem for us. (Note: To those who question this early introduction of meat, I point to the widely accepted, even earlier introduction of meats in prematures—a practice recommended by many eminent authorities on baby feeding.)

At 17 Days, Soups and Meat Combinations, such as lamb and rice or beef and vegetables, are introduced, and we realize now that baby is eating regular little meals. He may have meat and vegetable combinations and a milk feeding for dinner, or vegetables and meat separately; he might have soup and cereal at night, or meat and cereal at that time. It is highly desirable to keep away from stereotyped meals, to prevent baby's forming preferences. Can you think of anything more dull than being faced with the same foods or combination of foods several days in a row?

At 17-21 Days, eliminate the midnight feeding. At about three weeks the midnight feeding may be dropped, having fully served its purpose, which was not to pacify the infant but his parents, grandparents, neighbors and doubting friends. Many babies, to my knowledge, have gone without the midnight feeding either from birth or shortly thereafter with no untoward effects. I am often asked how a mother may know when her baby is ready to dispense with his midnight feeding, and I answer that when he is difficult to waken, or once having been roused refuses to take more than an ounce or so of milk or five minutes' breast feeding, he is signifying his own readiness.

At 3 Weeks, Fruit Juice. Each new addition to your baby's diet is an exciting event. Will he like it? Will it agree with him? Well, why not? Millions before him have eaten and digested the same foods, and it's reasonable to suppose that he will, also. Now, with the coming of his third week, the baby is introduced to fruit juice. Initially, he is offered orange juice combined with an equal amount of water as a part of his breakfast. This may be fresh, frozen or canned juice, any of which may have to be strained, not so much for baby's benefit as to keep nipples from clogging.

At 4 Weeks, Cod Liver Oil (Optional). Cod liver oil or other vitamin supplement may be added at about four weeks at the discretion of the supervising physician. I am inclined to feel that the use of these supplements is unnecessary, inasmuch as baby is already receiving adequate amounts of all the vitamins as well as the necessary minerals in his regular diet, if he is being fed according to this schedule. Your baby's doctor will advise you on this point.

At 5 Weeks, Eggs are introduced, and this addition provokes a great deal of controversial comment. Some authorities insist that baby must not be given anything but hard-boiled yolks despite the fact that they occasionally evoke gagging, spitting and vomiting. Interesting enough, feeding tests have shown that babies accepted and tolerate the commercially prepared strained egg yolks better than the hard-boiled yolks. In my practice, I have found that babies accept the whole egg far better than the yolk alone. An easy, palatable, and safe way of giving baby eggs is by offering them in a very soft scrambled state (softer than an adult would eat but not runny) which means that they must be prepared over a low flame or on the "medium" heat of an electric range. Too much heat will cause them to harden before you know it. At about eight weeks or so, coddled eggs may be given as an alternate to the soft scrambled ones.

We're gaining ground now, having added a number of items to milk, and before long we can add regular fruit to the ever-growing list. Not bad for such a little shaver.

At 6-8 Weeks, Fruits, Custards, Puddings. I can hear your next question—"When do we add fruits, custards, and puddings?"—almost as though we were sitting across the room talking to one another. This is a point at which I urge procrastination, if possible, for once added to a baby's diet sweet foods become—and remain—a problem. There is almost never any difficulty in the introduction of these foods, which, incidentally, should include the strained fruits and fresh bananas. A frequent reaction is for baby to rebel against acceptance of his plain foods once he has tasted the sweet ones. When mothers call me aghast at this development, I ask who's the bigger and smarter, baby or Mother? If baby is permitted to dictate at this point, a new pattern of food appreciation is set up and sweets take top billing when they should be last on the list. A positive, firm approach is the only one to take at this point.

At 9 Weeks, Bacon and Eggs, Just Like Dad! In not-so-strange logic, the use of bacon is included in the category of sweets. Whereas it is often necessary to advise mothers of ways and means to introduce the plainer meats, I cannot recall a single incident where the much coarser bacon has presented any problem, whether given alone or with egg. At nine weeks, prepared in the usual American manner with emphasis on the crispness, then cut finely and crumbled with a fork, the saltiness and bacony taste is most acceptable to baby. He loves it! You might occasionally try commercially prepared strained egg yolks and bacon, a tasty blend of egg yolks with a small amount of bacon that babies seem to enjoy so much.

The fact that I have neglected to mention certain vegetables and fruits does not mean that they must be omitted from the baby's diet. Keeping in mind the introduction dates for each type of food (vegetables at ten days; strained meats at fourteen days; fruit juices at three weeks; strained fruits at six weeks, etc.) you may offer beets, sweet potatoes and even corn (strained) as alternate vegetables, and peaches, pears, applesauce, bananas and prunes in the fruit category. Any strained food available in the grocery store may be given once the general classification of vegetables or fruit has been introduced. Rather than cover every detail of feeding in every phase of childhood, I think mothers can best judge for themselves, after baby has gotten beyond the first three months, when he's ready for another step toward eating like an adult. Recent years have seen the introduction of so-called "Junior" foods, which are not strained. Starting at about five months, baby can start on the regular adult foods, mashed at the table with the back of a fork. Highly spiced or exotic foods (fried shrimp, sausage, chili con carne, etc.) should be avoided at first, although youngsters in Italian-American families take to spaghetti and even pizza like ducks to water, starting as early as four or five months.

Solid Foods and Development. It has often been intimated, particularly by mothers whose babies develop rather rapidly, that my program of early introduction of solid foods has speeded up the development pattern as a whole. "After all," it is frequently argued, "Johnnie started eating meat and vegetables much earlier than most babies. Isn't it logical that he get over his 'baby' ways more quickly than average, and don't you think that accounts for his crawling so soon?"

After such questions had been posed a few times, I was interested enough to check into the matter. I checked on the ages of first teeth, first steps, and other events in a group of children who had been given solid foods early in life and compared the results with other youngsters. I could find no significant difference from the norm. In each group there were babies who developed rapidly and others who were slower, and I have therefore made no claim that my feeding program will cause babies to be smarter, quicker to develop, or otherwise achieve the milestones of infancy and childhood any more rapidly than other youngsters.

I do believe that there are definite advantages in the early introduction of solid foods, together with a general program that requires the baby to fit into the family routine rather than letting the family revolve around baby. These advantages are related to later life, however, and to better harmony between husband and wife while baby is still in infancy. This program was developed, you'll remember, because I am a family doctor primarily interested in seeing that the new baby doesn't unnecessarily disrupt the life patterns of a hitherto happy married couple. The marked advantages to the baby were not anticipated.

Smaller Appetite After First Year. Many mothers begin feeding their children between meals because they're afraid the child may not be getting enough to eat, especially if he isn't eating as much at mealtimes as he did earlier in life. What has really happened, of course, is that the baby has gotten over his initial period of very rapid growth and now needs less food than formerly. It isn't unusual for a perfectly normal baby to be eating only half as much at a year as he was at six months—although many mothers are simply horrified at this development.

"But, Doctor, he eats so little," is a complaint I often hear. When I check into the matter, I almost invariably find that the reduced food intake is adequate for the current growth rate; any additional food would merely cause him to become more chubby than I like to see. As when he was an infant, the one-year-old should be fed at mealtimes and not between. If he doesn't eat, he simply isn't hungry and can wait until the next meal.

By the first birthday, and preferably earlier, every child should have a portion of each food the family is eating for a particular meal. More often than not, table food will be all he'll need, although in certain situations the family's main course may be too spicy or too exotic for the baby. In such cases he should have a little taste of adult food, supplemented by something made especially for him (a jar of Junior food, perhaps), together with potatoes and vegetabes from the table. In this way, he learns to eat everything and to appreciate foods other than his favorites.

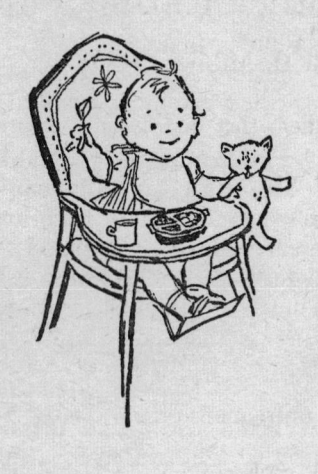

Toddler Eating Patterns

by Elizabeth D. Munves, Ph.D.

THE toddler—that cuddlesome combination of contradictions—often causes his mother unnecessary worry. Rapid changes in growth and development take place from the time a baby begins to walk until he is about three. Many parents are alarmed at such normal patterns as a sharp decrease in appetite and refusal of "good" foods, like milk.

The nutritive needs of the year-older and up—the amounts of vitamins, minerals, proteins and calories—are related to his physical growth. But the food he eats to supply those nutrients is often dictated by his emotional growth.

As usual, each child is an individual and many of these variations were decided for him before he was born. Heredity determines many physical characteristics and family background influences the foods on the dinner table. Recognition and understanding of his changing from a dependent baby to an independent one year old is an important help in developing healthy attitudes towards food.

The physical development of the toddler is markedly different from that of the infant. Sometimes a mother does not notice that the rate of growth of her baby has slowed down as he neared his first birthday. As a toddler, his arms and legs will grow more rapidly than his trunk.

At a year and a half there occurs a surge of growth in the skeletal musculature. This rapid muscle growth continues throughout the toddler age. In fact, it has been shown that about ½ of the child's total weight gain from 1½ to 3 years is due to growth of muscle.

Other changes occur in the skeleton. Its growth rate has decreased, similar to that of the total body growth, and therefore, it has slowed down. But, an important point, minerals are being deposited at an increased rate, so that the skeleton, while not growing in length, becomes stronger.

It is during this period that the toddler loses his baby fat and replaces it with larger amounts of muscle. Thus, even in appearance, mothers see their "baby" changing into a child. Shifts in water content of the toddler's body also contribute to his over-all growth. During this period the content of his body water decreases and more of it is found inside the muscle cells.

Nutritively, then, the toddler has increased demands for the "raw" material for muscular and skeletal growth and development. Authorities believe that hereditary factors determine a child's potential for growth but that unless he receives the amount of nutrients needed at each stage, he cannot maintain his own individual rate of growth. As a result, it is possible that he may arrive at the next age with a deficit.

There are, of course, many psychological changes within the child during this toddler period that can affect his food intake. The wise mother recognizes these and tries to avoid their becoming serious blocks to eating. The toddler frequently finds mealtime a good time to assert his independence. He wants to do things for himself, even if it means dropping foods on the floor. It is a laughing and lovable age which can quickly change to tears if frustrations occur. His desire to help and his tendency for imitation can be effectively used in developing desirable attitudes towards foods. All mothers are aware that it is the toddler who discovers the meaning and power of "no."

The nutrients that receive special emphasis in the toddler's requirements are protein, calcium, phosphorus, and calories. Other vitamins and minerals are not forgotten, of course, but usually the necessary amounts of these nutrients are provided in the foods that supply the high protein needs.

Protein is necessary for normal rapid muscle growth as well as the growth of other body tissues. A toddler should have approximately a gram and a half of protein for each pound of weight. As a basis for comparison, a man requires ½ gram of protein for each pound of weight. Thus, the toddler's need is three times that of an adult. At least half of the protein should come from animal sources: meats, milk, fish, poultry, cheese and eggs. The remainder may be supplied by vegetable sources such as peas, beans and cereals and breads.

On the average, the protein requirement will increase from 35 grams per day at one year, to 40 at two and to 45 grams per day at three years. These can easily be provided by one to one and a half pints of milk (16 to 24 grams of protein), an egg (7 grams), 1 ounce (2 tbsp. either ground or small pieces) of meat, fish or poultry, (7 grams), 3 slices of bread, whole grain or enriched (6 grams), and 1 serving of cereal (2 grams). Protein may also be supplied in small amounts (approximately 2 grams in each serving) by vegetables. An ounce of hard cheese or cottage cheese can provide approximately the same amount of protein as meat.

Because of the strengthening of bones, calcium and phosphorus deserve special attention in the toddler's diet. This requirement is met by the one to one and a half pints of milk mentioned previously. The child also needs sufficient vitamin D, 300-400 units, to insure retention of calcium and phosphorus.

The boundless energy of the toddler amazes most

mothers. "Surely" they think, "he must need loads of calories to keep going like that from morning to night!" Surprisingly, the caloric needs are not high, and they increase very slowly from ages one to three. It is true that once he has begun to walk (and run!) the baby needs more calories for activity. But he needs fewer calories for general growth. Various studies have shown that a child may need approximately 1,025 calories when he is a year old. This may increase by as little as 275 calories, up to 1,300, by his third birthday.

Caloric needs will vary from child to child. Some children are relatively quiet, being content to play in the sand box, while a contemporary will spend his time climbing the steps to the slide. As is true in the adult, a larger child with greater muscular development will expend more calories at the same task than a smaller youngster.

Also, a child's caloric needs will vary from day to day. The energy expended on a rainy day in the house may be less than one spent outside. The toddler's appetite is a fairly reliable guide to his caloric needs.

Other nutrients are usually found in the foods mentioned previously. Iron is provided from many sources: eggs, meats, green leafy vegetables and enriched breads and cereals. However, only small amounts of iron are found in each of these foods. Consequently it is important to include some of each of these in the diet. Vitamin A is found in egg, whole milk, liver, butter and margarine, and vitamin A value is provided by green leafy and yellow vegetables.

Thiamine is another nutrient that is found in small amounts in many foods. The toddler will get his supply from meats, egg and enriched breads and cereals. Potatoes, especially cooked in the jacket, will provide some thiamine. Milk is a rich source of riboflavin, another of the B vitamins. Other B vitamins may be supplied by egg, meat, enriched or whole grain breads and cereals and vegetables. Vitamin C needs will be met by a serving of citrus fruit. During the summer months, servings of other fresh fruits, as the toddler grows older and can eat them, will provide vitamin C.

Foods that should be avoided in the toddler's diet fall into two groups; those that he cannot handle and thereby are potential hazards, and the foods considered as unnecessary. The former consist of foods that contain seeds or pits, such as cherries, grapes, nuts, gristle around bone, and bites of tough fruit skin. These items can be too easily inhaled. Many fruits can be pitted and peeled to avoid this difficulty.

Sweet foods, such as sugar, candy, frostings, syrups, soft drinks, and jams and jellies should not be included in the diet of the toddler. There are many reasons for this. A toddler has a limited capacity for food, and these items which contain only calories can displace foods that are needed for vitamin and mineral content as well as calories. Sweets depress a child's appetite, thus diminishing his desire for other foods. Even when these items are offered at the end of a meal, they are often given in the form of a reward. This can create an undesirable attitude about their place in the diet. And, finally, parents need always to keep in mind that they are developing food habits to last a lifetime. The role of unnecessary sweet foods in the dental health of the individual and the part that sweets play in the food patterns of many overweight children and adults is too well recognized today to ignore. There are, of course, special occasions, like birthday parties, where tradition temporarily overrules common sense.

Mothers often forget that emotional reactions to food are usually temporary. Children, especially the toddler, pass through a variety of eating phases. At one time, they may eat anything in sight, and the next day cut down to almost nothing. At other times they may eat one food to the exclusion of another. Usually these food jags are of short duration and are harmless as long as only good nutritious foods are provided.

Often a toddler is not satisfied with the usual three meals. He needs to eat more often, so his snacks should be such foods as fruit, graham crackers, small servings of milk; part of the daily diet. Small portions are usually enough for the toddler. Dawdlers are common, and if he is in the process of learning to feed himself, he may need a little help. Many children are too hungry and too tired to wait until the family dinner hour. All of these individual points should be recognized and the child fed accordingly. It is important that no issue develop over eating to color a youngsters pleasure in food in future years.

Although the toddler's nutritional needs are high, it is possible to meet them with easy-to-get, inexpensive foods. It is equally desirable to develop cooperation with the toddler as he learns to feed himself and select his foods. Occasionally parents need to examine their own food patterns to be certain that these are the ones they want their children to imitate. After all, the apple doesn't fall far from the tree!

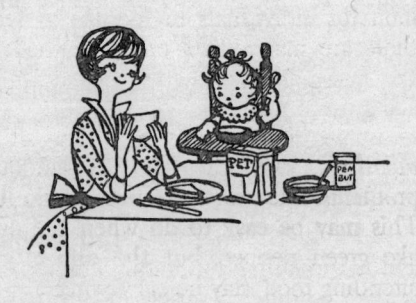

Food Allergies

by Elizabeth D. Munves, Ph.D.

MANY mothers have children who are allergic to certain foods. And these mothers have questions concerning food selection and food preparation. They want to know how to plan menus that omit these foods and they want to know where they can obtain information about recipes omitting certain key foods. We realized that these are real problems to many mothers when we received a large number of letters following an article about food allergies.

A food allergy can be detected only through painstaking investigation by a physician. It has become common for individuals to indulge in self-diagnosis so that there are many diets omitting foods unnecessarily. So, the first point to keep in mind is: Be sure that your allergy is a true one.

Once a particular food or a list of foods has been identified, then the cook in the family has constant problems. She has to cut out certain items from the diet. This may be easy to do when the culprit is something like green pepper, but the difficulty occurs when the offending food may be eggs, wheat, or milk—foods which might be considered staples of our diet. Not only do these foods appear on the table singly, such as poached eggs, shredded wheat or a glass of milk, but they often are used in the preparation of other items. Apart from obvious combinations like cake and mayonnaise, eggs appear in other unsuspected foods like some candies, glazings for coffee cake and noodles. The alert mother has to literally become a detective. One of her most reliable clues in avoiding the allergen is information appearing on the food label itself.

Fortunately many of the items that may need to be eliminated are in the category known to nutritionists as "extra foods." Those that provide mainly calories, such as cake, cookies and candy can be left out of the diet for the child without jeopardizing his health. The calories can be provided from other sources. However, since youngsters do like treats, other forms of these foods can be provided as substitutes.

When a mother is given a list of foods to avoid, the foods often seem to have no relationship to one another. One such list that a reader submitted to us and asked for help in planning included the following items: eggs, barley, lemon, grapefruit, grape, chocolate, fowl, fish. Thus, the most logical step is to begin with menu planning. But all concerned must keep in mind that substitutes are not duplicates of the replaced foods. These duplications should not be compared unfavorably to the replaced food.

Nutritionists are accustomed to planning menus on the basis of Four Food Groups. So, when there is any change in the foods allowed, it is simplest to adjust within these groups.

Meat group. We need two or more servings per day of any meat, fish or poultry. Eggs can be considered as an occasional meat substitute. Many readers wrote to say that their children were allergic to certain meats—but none mentioned to *all* meats. So, if fish or chicken has to be omitted, then other meats can be selected. Whenever chicken, for example, is served to the family, then another kind of meat should be offered to the allergic one. This is not spoiling!

Eggs, however, are not so easily avoided. They are basic to the preparation of many foods, cakes, pie fillings, cookies, muffins, pancakes and many other favorite items. Some of these foods can be prepared without eggs, though the product is not quite the same. Perhaps the doctor can tell if a child is allergic to the whole egg or to the yolk or the white. If either of the latter can be used, there is greater leeway in cooking. From a nutritional standpoint, we depend upon the yolk for its iron and protein content. The white provides protein. Liver is an excellent source of iron and the B vitamins usually supplied by the egg and can be included in the diet weekly.

Milk group. Children need 3 to 4 cups daily or its equivalent in cheese (not cream cheese) products. We depend upon this group to provide calcium, protein and riboflavin. Many readers indicated that they needed to omit milk from children's diets. If the doctor permits, the soy bean milks that are available are adequate nutritional substitutes. Companies which make these also have recipe booklets containing recipes for using soy bean milk in many prepared foods which mothers can request. Because a child uses milk each meal, it is difficult to substitute any but the soy bean milk. Children soon become quite fond of it, even if the taste is strange at first.

Vegetable and fruit group. This should include a citrus fruit or other fruit or vegetable important for vitamin C, a dark green or deep-yellow vegetable (at least every other day), and one or two servings of other fruits and vegetables, including potatoes. From the letters received, almost every item in this category is suspect for some child. However, substitutions are usually easy to find, even though the substitute may be an unfamiliar vegetable to the child. If he's allergic to spinach (most children would tell you they are if given the chance), kale can be easily substituted. Foods like bananas, cucumber and string beans can be omitted and others served.

Citrus fruits, which provide the major source of our vitamin C, are more difficult to replace, nutrition-wise. If oranges need to be omitted, then other citrus fruits, grapefruit, tangerines, or tomatoes will supply vitamin C. The portions should be a little larger. Fresh fruits in season, such as cantaloupe, strawberries, and fresh vegetables, especially raw ones, like green pepper, contain vitamin C.

Bread and cereal group: (whole grain, enriched, or restored). 4 or more servings each day. These are significant sources of the B vitamins and iron, and of some protein. Wheat is among the most common food allergens and one that appears in many prepared foods. The structure of wheat protein expands so that when bread rises it is the wheat that helps it to hold its shape and be called a "light" dough. Thus, while it is common knowledge that our bread is made from wheat, it is not so well known that it is also an ingredient in corn bread, rye bread and other types. Practically all noodles, spaghetti and macaroni as well as crackers are made from wheat.

This is the most difficult group of all to substitute. A leisurely trip to the supermarket when the shopper can take time to carefully read labels on boxes will reveal many cereals that do not contain wheat: these are corn and rye products. Recipes on the boxes will give suggestions for preparing cookies and snacks for the wheat-allergic child. Letters to these companies may also bring other dishes.

One reader indicated that she needed a recipe for non-allergic bread. Since many mothers need a similar recipe, the following is included:

100% Rye Flour Bread

(No Wheat, Milk or Egg)

1 cake fresh yeast	4 teaspoons brown sugar
1¼ cups lukewarm water	4 cups rye flour
1 teaspoon salt	

Dissolve yeast in ¼ cup lukewarm water. Mix with salt, sugar, and rest of water. Stir in flour, continue beating until dough is smooth. Turn out onto rye floured board. Then knead, add enough additional rye flour (if necessary) to make a firm, elastic dough. Place in greased bowl, brush top with salad oil, cover and let rise in warm place until double in bulk. Knead a second time, and then place in bowl and let rise again (approx. 1 hour). Shape into loaf and place in greased 9" × 5" × 3" loaf pan. Cover with clean towel, let rise in warm place until double in bulk. Bake in hot oven (450 F) for 15 minutes, then reduce heat to 350 and finish baking (about 45 to 50 minutes).

There are many individuals and organizations to whom mothers with allergic children may turn for help. Ask the doctor if he thinks there is a dietitian at his hospital who may be able to help with making dietary substitutions. (Not all hospitals are fortunate enough to have such trained personnel).

The American Dietetic Association, 620 N. Michigan Avenue, Chicago, Illinois, 60611 is another source of help. Two kinds of information may be obtained here. An allergy booklet containing wheat, egg and milk-free recipes prepared by its members is available for 50 cents a copy. You might also ask them if there is a District Dietetic Association in your area or some individual who might help plan menus. Perhaps someone nearby is a dietitian-turned-homemaker.

The home economist in the agricultural extension program may be able to suggest ways of preparing foods without ingredients that are usually considered essential. If she cannot help you, she is probably aware of other sources. Another place for help is your state Department of Health. The nutritionist assigned to local areas knows how to adjust all allergy diets.

Foods that are free of common allergens are found at health food stores in most large cities. However, these items are expensive. It is more practical to write directly to a company, such as The Chicago Dietetic Supply House, Inc., 1750 West Van Buren, Chicago, Illinois, 60612 for a catalogue and price list. Ask for dietary products for allergy diets.

While it is unfortunate that a child has to do without certain foods for a time, mothers should guard against adopting an "I'm so sorry for you" attitude. Equally important is to avoid a resentful feeling about the extra bother this creates. Allergic reactions are usually so difficult to detect that it is indeed fortunate if the doctor has determined that certain foods are causing that nasty rash —and it may be only for a short while!

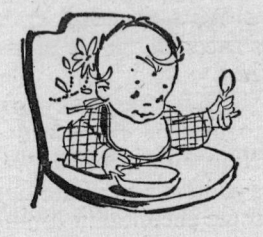

Allergies (Other Than Foods)

by Elliot F. Ellis, M.D.

ALLERGIES, the most common chronic illness among children, often affect babies during the first weeks of their life. Indeed, a large proportion of the one in ten Americans who has an allergy began life with a cough or an itch or another of the many signs of this galaxy of diseases. Particularly if there is a history of allergy in your family, you should know about this condition and what to do about it.

To begin, just what is an allergy? A popular definition might be this: It is the sensitivity of a person to a substance that is usually harmless to other people. The substance can be a pollen that affects his nose and results in hay fever. It can be an irritant to the skin that brings on eczema. It can affect the bronchial tubes and cause the most serious of allergies, asthma.

There are many kinds of allergies, and even more substances that can cause them. These substances, called allergens, may include in addition to pollens, such substances in the air as mold spores, insect dust or house dust.

They may also include household chemicals such as room deodorizers or dyes, drugs such as aspirin or penicillin, animal dander, soap, insect stings or feathers. Even a mother's perfume can bring on an allergic reaction if some chemical in it proves irritating to baby's system.

Parents often believe that foods cause a great many allergies. Foods such as eggs, milk or cereal certainly do cause some allergies, it is true, but they are greatly overrated as allergens.

In fact, in two medical papers delivered at the American Academy of Allergy meeting earlier this year it was shown that foods cause fewer allergies in children than they are commonly believed to.

Regardless of what may be causing an allergy, what is important for a parent to know is whether or not a child has an allergy. If baby has a persistent night cough, it can be an early sign of a respiratory allergy such as asthma. Shortness of breath or rapid breathing can also be signs of respiratory allergies. Sometimes the condition will come and go and sometimes it will be continual; in either event if baby has these symptoms you should have him examined by your physician.

Similarly, if baby keeps rubbing or scratching his face, arms or legs, or the creases in his body, this might mean he has a skin allergy like infantile eczema. One of the more common skin allergies among babies, infantile eczema often begins very early in life. Usually it disappears when the child reaches three to five years of age, but sometimes it becomes a chronic condition. In this case, the patient's skin becomes thickened, bringing not only discomfort but also personality problems for many persons.

Indeed, allergies of all types have a way of worsening and becoming chronic. In addition, one allergy can easily lead to another, usually a more serious one. For these reasons it is important for parents to recognize symptoms as soon as possible and to get medical attention if they have allergies.

It is especially important for children in families with a history of allergy to have medical attention. These children are more likely than others to develop serious allergies. For example, a baby with eczema whose parents both have asthma is twice as likely to have asthma as a baby with eczema but without a family history of asthma.

Research at National Jewish Hospital at Denver demonstrates that children with allergies, even chronic allergies like asthma, can lead happy and healthy lives with the proper medical treatment. The hospital, a free, non-sectarian center for all chronic chest diseases specializes in the care of children with very severe, chronic asthma. Most of its patients who are admitted have been treatment failures in their home communities and are sent to National Jewish Hospital as sort of a last resort.

Doctors treating allergy patients begin the course of treatment in much the same way a detective begins his investigation at the scene of a crime, by looking for clues. While the detective combs the scene for tell-tale signs that will lead to the culprit, the allergist begins a methodical search for the identity of the allergen causing the illness.

He will investigate the family history, the frequency and the timing of episodes of the illness, their complications, places visited prior to episodes, etc. Parents who keep a "diary" of the circumstances surrounding each attack will help the doctor in his search for the allergen.

When he has narrowed down his list of suspects, the doctor may check the guilt of each one with an allergy skin test. The test consists of scratching a liquid form of the suspected allergen onto the skin of the child's arm or back. If a positive reaction develops, this allergen may be a cause of the illness. A variation of the scratch is the intradermal test, where the suspected allergen is injected under the patient's skin rather than scratched on.

It should be noted that these tests are not foolproof and that they can give misleading results. This is particularly true with food allergens, which are harder to test for than airborne allergens. The doctor may thus want to supplement these tests with others.

One of these additional tests commonly used with

babies is what is called the "passive transfer test." In this case, the doctor injects serum from the baby's body into the skin of a volunteer and gives the volunteer an intradermal test at that spot 48 hours later. Sometimes doctors will use this passive transfer test as the first test in small infants and children who because of skin conditions or lack of cooperation cannot be tested directly.

There are still more ways to identify the offending allergen. Whatever the test used, the doctor will test its conclusions by purposely exposing the patient to the allergen in its natural form and noting his response. Once he is satisfied he has identified the allergen or allergens, he will tell the parents how they can help the child avoid the cause of the allergy.

If the allergen is dust, the parents may be advised to remove dust-collectors from the child's room. The doctor may suggest installing an air filter that collects pollens or mold spores by electrical attraction. If animal danders are to blame you may have to give the family pet away.

Try as you might, it is sometimes difficult to eliminate the allergens from the child's environment. In those cases the doctor may advise trying to immunize the child against his allergy's causes. He will inject minute amounts of the allergen into the bloodstream over a period of time in the hope of preparing the body to deal with the allergen effectively.

In addition to immunizing "shots", in the case of asthma, the doctor may prescribe drugs that help the child breathe more easily and keep attacks under control. These drugs must be used with great care, for they often have undesirable side-effects.

Doctors are making substantial progress in the fight against allergies. As the experience at National Jewish Hospital indicates, the patient today has a better chance than ever of living a full and happy life.

SECTION V

Personality and Emotional Development

Sibling Rivalry

by **Alfred J. Vignec, M.D.**

MANY people feel that in this modern day when so much is said about sibling rivalry it has almost ceased to be a problem. One very successful young mother of three small children recently intimated to me that it belongs to the dark ages when nothing was known about child psychology, and that it is almost pointless to discuss it in these enlightened times. Parents have learned to avoid the pitfalls, and guide family relationships into the proper channels.

It is true that in some families there is little or no jealousy or envy between brother and sister, and a feeling of general unity prevails. This is, of course, the ideal. However, the other picture is all too familiar—one child enjoys seeing the other punished, one hates the other's successes, there is too much competition for attention, and arguing and quarrelling reach disturbing proportions. Parents often take sides in such situations and strong favoritisms may develop.

As is usual with all problems of this type, it is far better and easier to attempt to prevent intense rivalry between siblings than to deal with it once it has developed. Prevention must begin at the outset.

Preparation of the small child for the arrival of the new baby begins as soon as the mother realizes that she is pregnant. Children under two or over six usually adjust

SIBLING RIVALRY

readily and welcome the baby into the home with little or no traumatic reaction. The infant under two is pliable as a rule, and able to accept a change in the family set-up. The child of school age feels mature and far removed from the world of infancy and its needs. He is not likely to long for the type of attention the baby receives; he feels superior to its helplessness and falls naturally into the role of guide and protector. It is very flattering to have a baby clutch his finger and copy his actions.

Children between two and five years of age are most likely to feel resentment and envy. Also, the two-child group, while it exists, is usually the most difficult. One child has had stage center and must relinquish it and share. Future additions are less distressing. Even in later life, the two eldest in a family may compete most strongly.

On the other hand, if the mother is careful and affectionate, the new baby and his 2-5 year old sibling may be very happy together. Most important of all, the older child must not be made to feel that the baby is an intruder who has come to take from him some of his parents' affection, his toys, his prized possessions, the familiarity of his precious little rituals—even his crib. The removal from the crib should be accomplished during the first few months of the mother's pregnancy, and no mention should be made of using it for the baby. Emphasis should be placed solely on the fact that a bed is "grown up", and it should be built up as a pleasant accomplishment to be allowed to have one. Almost every baby loves his crib and regards it as a haven of safety and security, and the thought that it is to be given to another may cause considerable shock and hostility. The new baby should be referred to as "ours" even before it arrives, and the older child should be told how much the baby will love him. Occasionally, a mother is somewhat startled by being told quite frankly, "I don't want a baby. Don't get one". In such cases it is best not to press the point too strongly, but to be affectionate and warm to the child, and hope for a change in attitude when the newcomer actually appears.

Once the baby has arrived, it is very difficult for the mother, still somewhat exhausted from the ordeal of the birth, burdened with new duties, and face to face with the pressing business of rearranging her routine, to give as much time and attention to the older child as previously. Also, a new baby is always "cute" to outsiders, and the older child will suffer a little from this, however well prepared. In time, though, he may feel flattered himself when the smaller one is complimented, if he loves it, takes pride in it and feels it is partly his.

The mother is wise to be very cautious about singing the same songs to the baby, using the same pet-names, or giving the baby favorite and recognizable toys, unless the older child is willing. Also, remember how important familiar routines are to the older child (mealtime, bathtime, naptime and bedtime procedures, etc.) and avoid changing them suddenly, so that the child feels he has lost something by the baby's arrival.

Emphasize maturity ("You're a big boy now, helping Mommy,"; "You can show baby sister how to do things," etc.), but don't expect him to grow up too quickly, or lose patience with his infantile mannerisms. In fact, you may well expect more to develop—a return to the bottle, a desire to eat some of the baby's strained foods, even a wish to put on diapers, at least in play. Nursery school teachers often notice that, after the arrival of a new baby in the home, a three year old girl insists on being the baby in household play situations, when before she had always eagerly awaited her turn to be the "Mommy."

Helping with the new baby is very beneficial, although it can be dangerous, as the small child can easily overestimate his ability. Hence, the mother must be on constant guard against mishaps. One mother discovered her 4-year-old "giving the baby a bath"—another was shocked to find the 3-week-old baby missing from his crib and eventually found her 3-year-old wheeling him around in the doll carriage.

In general, the small child who has had good relations with his parents (especially the mother) will accept the arrival of the new baby quite satisfactorily. However, tact and affection must continuously be used, during early childhood particularly, to guard against a rupture in the relationship.

Perhaps the most important thing is to permit him to have his own way when possible. Each of us has likes and dislikes. We all want to assert ourselves. If the matter is not important, let him win. On the other hand, if he is refusing to do something which should or must be done, simply be firm and proceed despite his protests, at the same time explaining to him why it must be done, and that there are times when he may do as he wishes and other times when that is impossible. Many little ones appreciate explanations, even at an early age. Above all, they get a sense of fairness when they are allowed to do as they wish at least part of the time. But be consistent in your attitude. Don't take a stand unless you have to, but once you have taken it, see it through.

At times if his "no" is simply ignored, he will do the accepted thing, even after protest. For example, the best management for the little boy who refuses what his mother offers and then asks for the same thing is to just accept his "no's" and then give him his apple and toast as though the whole thing had been his own idea.

On occasion, if the "no" is a particularly ridiculous one, it is quite acceptable to treat it with humor. If the child can be made to join in and laugh at himself, it is an excellent treatment. One little fellow picked up a book for his father, and this conversation followed. "Thank you. That's a good boy." "No, I'm not a good boy". Daddy smiled. "Are you a naughty boy?" "No, I'm not a naughty boy". "Are you a boy?" "No, I'm not a boy". "Are you a girl, then"? "No, I'm not a girl." "Well, if you're not a boy and not a girl, you must be a puppy dog. Hello, there, puppy dog." This was greeted by a burst of laughter from the family, in which the two-year-old was the most enthusiastic participant. At times, after this incident, when asked "Are you a good boy?" he would answer, "No, I'm a puppy dog," and wait for the expected laughter, in which he again would join happily. So long as the child is not made a fool of, embarrassed, or laughed at unkindly, humor has a definite value in child management. Most children like to laugh—if they can be amused by themselves (and also amuse others) they develop tolerance and good-nature.

Distraction is usually an excellent aid in the management of negativism, as in the management of many other behavior situations involving small children. It might be almost called the parents' best single strategy. It will not always work, of course, but it frequently helps. If the child's attention is directed to something else, very often he forgets he has said "no", and the crisis is avoided.

Above all, though, constant argument is fatal. If the little one feels that he will always be talked down, that his ideas and opinions and inclinations are of no importance, that a stronger voice will be raised against him, no matter what he says, he is well on the way to becoming a chronic no-sayer throughout childhood. Instead of a harmless and normal method of self-expression, "no" becomes a weapon against his mother and the world. He uses it to defy and defeat adults and other children. It is his method of revenge and retribution. And he has acquired a problem which will then have to be approached with understanding and patience if his confidence in the rightness of things is to be restored.

But the two-year-old who has been tactfully handled during this trying early negativism "grows out of it" quite spontaneously. In time he becomes bored with it all. Growth brings new interests and new maturity. His mastery of different objects, his wider vistas of thought and action give him fresh fields to conquer and other goals to seek. He may betray his change of interest initially by saying "no" as usual, then hesitating for a minute and saying "yes", quite naturally, and without adult prompting. This "no-yes" period is the mother's first welcome sign that another hurdle has been crossed and left behind.

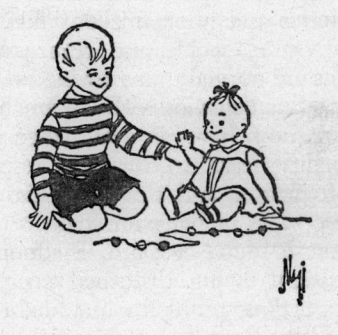

Your Baby's Behavior

by Walter J. Coville, Ph.D.

YOUR baby's initial adjustments to the outside world are instinctive and unorganized. Thus, he may cry, sleep fitfully, sneeze, suckle and regurgitate his food. These reactions are normal in a growing infant and most mothers accept this behavior without much concern. As the child grows, he behaves in accordance with his own unique personality, learning from and responding characteristically to people and things in his environment. However, some types of behavior shake a mother's confidence and cause much concern. Predominant among these are persistent crying, disturbed sleep, thumbsucking, temper tantrums, problems in toilet training, fears and other manifestations of instability.

Crying: This is a child's normal expression of hunger, discomfort, fear or his need to have mother's attention, especially at night. Generally, it is better in these circumstances to limit the amount of attention you give him. Later, the growing baby cries to express anger and other related emotions. Here, pampering must be avoided, since it only leads to excessive demands by means of crying and whining. An understanding but firm and secure approach by you will prevent the development of a serious crying problem.

Sleeping: Newborn infants sleep most of the time, awakening only for feeding or when disturbed. The very young child should sleep as long as he wants to. (The child of age 2 averages one awakening per night, whereas at age 3 he usually sleeps through the entire night.) Sleeping time should be as regular as possible. Threats and emotional scenes disturb the child's sleep and when problems develop, they are manifested by irregular sleeping habits, nightmares or bed-wetting. Poor training, over-protection, pampering, or parental fears may be causes of sleep disturbance. Treatment should include an evaluation of your own role in this problem; sleeping patterns should be regular; the attitude in the home should be calm and reassuring.

Thumbsucking: In a very young child, thumbsucking satisfies a real need and is a natural activity. Experts estimate that about 25% of all children develop this habit early, and it may continue up to age 4. However, mothers become concerned since they fear that oral deformities will result. Dentists, however, seriously question this. Mothers also feel that this habit constitutes "bad manners" and reflects their inefficient training. Thumbsucking is a source of pleasure and security to the infant and an issue should not be made of it. It may be a response to hunger, too early or abrupt weaning, loneliness, or feelings of neglect or insecurity. It is generally agreed that a direct attack on this habit by means of mechanical restraints, parental nagging and use of bitter tasting applications is undesirable. Such methods only aggravate the problem.

Temper tantrums: These include violent outbursts of anger with loss of control, screaming, kicking or breath-holding. In infancy, they may be set off by hampered movements or by sudden interruption of any satisfying and pleasurable activity. In dealing with temper tantrums, the mother must remain calm and avoid bribes or giving in to the child since this will encourage repetition. In severe instances, remove the child from the scene and avoid touching or caressing him. If necessary, a tepid bath may help. An atmosphere of serenity, self-control and the avoidance of attention-getting scenes (such as those that occur at feedings) will help prevent tantrums.

Toilet training: Most children establish bowel control by age 2 and bladder control by age 3, but in all instances, training should be begun when the child is ready. Usually training begins at about seven to twelve months. Problems in training are due to physical and psychological causes. Threats, bribes, coercion for very early training, as well as reactions of impatience and disappointment on the part of mother promote such problems. Training should be relaxed, unhurried, and in an atmosphere of understanding and support.

Fears and Emotional Instability: Many common fears arise in babyhood and the causes are varied. Sometimes these are unwittingly caused by parents, since even very young babies are suggestible and learn quickly. Other manifestations of instability or nervousness may be reactions to the environment. When such problems arise, they should be dealt with seriously since the fear is very real to the child.

Problem behavior in infants calls for skillful handling by the mother. A calm, loving, reassuring and supporting parent provides an atmosphere of security that in itself is the best preventive against the development of behavior problems.

Many parents regard such behavior as the desire for a pacifier, occasional refusals to eat or take the bottle, clinging to the mother, fear of visitors and similar patterns as "problem" behavior. Actually, there is no evidence of difficulty or poor adjustment in any of these activities; they are all normal manifestations of behavior at a certain stage of growth, and should be treated as such.

It is important to remember that babies are individuals and that no two are alike. Thus, behavior patterns will differ according to the temperament and personality of each child.

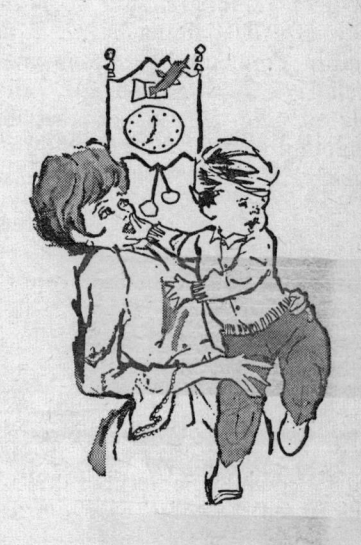

Habits—Good and Bad

by Alfred J. Vignec, M.D.

THE formation of acceptable habits in the baby and young child is extremely important. In the habit pattern lies the key to a happy childhood, a good parent-child relationship, and a well-adjusted adult personality. It's only a matter of how the acceptable patterns can be instilled successfully. Certainly not by force, nor the indiscriminate use of the hickory switch. More and more we have become aware that the baby is an individual with a will of his own, likes, dislikes, and preferences which he will uphold, often with a valiant struggle, if opposed. The more opposition, the greater the struggle, until at times an entire family can be set at odds by an "unruly" and self-willed child. Sometimes it is a very small child.

When the baby enters our world, he is faced by an alarming number of new facts to assimilate and problems to cope with. The amount of learning he does during his first year is really phenomenal. Some of this involves acquainting himself with the physical world of sights, odors, sounds, etc.; however, most of what he learns in some way involves other people—principally the mother.

In learning, he needs guidance. He is unable to use his own judgment, although he may often attempt to make decisions (usually the wrong ones). The world is filled with tempting objects, many of which are unsafe for him to touch and handle. His normal urges are interfered with by our codes of cleanliness and our cultural patterns and customs. Freedom for the baby would mean lapping up whatever food he wanted, salting at will, fingering and mouthing whatever he could lay his hands on, smashing things, staying up until he felt like sleeping, running about naked, etc. Of course, such conduct is impossible. He must be taught to conform, and as painlessly as possible.

The one positive factor which the mother and all caretakers have in teaching satisfactory habit patterns is that, initially, the baby wants to please. He thrives on praise and approval. He dislikes being shut out of the adult's good graces. This is understandable enough when one considers how dependent he is upon them. He needs them, loves them. He is happy when the relationship is smooth and undisturbed. On the other hand, he has his own basic urges and at a very early age wants his own way. It is up to the mother to make pleasing and conforming to the rules more desirable without unduly restricting his personality development.

How is this to be accomplished? Any teaching at all, especially at an early age, depends greatly on repetition for its effectiveness. It may seem ridiculous to the mother to repeat an action or a request ten or fifteen times a day, calmly and routinely, but at times this is necessary. It might almost be said that repetition is the secret of all early child training. Just as vital to success is patience. Every time the mother permits herself to be riled, or loses her temper in the course of training she loses ground. Calmness and gentleness woo the baby over to her side, and more than half of the struggle is won. It is also very important always to place emphasis on the positive rather than the negative. Praise for accomplishment rather than blaming for failure. This will be easier for the mother to do if she remembers that the *natural* thing for the baby to do is *not* to conform. Conforming involves learning and for a very little one such learning is difficult. Everyone who has handled children knows, however, that it is almost impossible to cope with a small child in adult surroundings without the judicious use of "no-no." It may frustrate him to be forbidden to handle pins and turn on the gas stove, but it may also save his life. If "no-no" is said cheerfully it does no harm, especially if the baby is praised when he is obedient. Many a little one will say "no-no" to himself when he passes a forbidden object, as if to remind himself of his mother's instructions.

The mother should expect failures, and not be discouraged by them. They are steps in the process of growth and development. Goals for babies and small children should not be set too high, as then genuine frustration follows. If too much direct opposition is used—scolding, punishment for small offenses, shaming and general disapproval—the baby is very likely to rebel, either subtly or openly. If the mother reacts with increased severity, a conflict develops. The baby no longer aims primarily to please. His motives are distorted. He now wants to defeat the mother. He is not old enough nor wise enough to guess at the reasons for his actions, but his behavior patterns follow a given course nevertheless. On the other hand, overly lenient handling is no better. If the baby lacks guidance, he also stands alone, not moving together with his mother but self-willed and at the same time insecure.

Many of a baby's early habit patterns seem to be part of his basic personality. There are major individual differences in temperament and approach even within the same family. Some babies are thumb suckers, some never try. Some tend to sleep a great deal while others require little sleep and resist naps vigorously. Some eat well, others poorly. Only within limits can such things be controlled. It is unwise to forcibly overstuff a "picky" eater, confine the active baby to his crib for long hours in a hopeless attempt to "make" him sleep, etc. All efforts by the mother should be made persistently, calmly, firmly

HABITS—GOOD AND BAD

but with judgment. Again let me emphasize the value of praise. Any child will obey more readily for love than to avoid discipline. This does not imply that discipline is without value, especially when the child emerges from infancy. There are many kinds, some good, some of dubious value or even harmful.

Nothing has been said regarding the distasteful habits that plague many mothers—such as thumbsucking, nail biting, nose picking, masturbation, chronic resistance to sleep and many others. While space does not permit detailed discussion at this time, let me say that these habits, especially if carried to extremes, are often emotional in origin and, if forcibly curtailed, may break out in another direction. An effort should be made to determine the cause and correct it, if possible. With regard to many of the minor "bad" habits of infancy, if the mother thinks back carefully she can often recall when and how the habit began—what was said or done to give rise to it, whom the baby copies, etc. Such habits, especially when traceable, can best be broken by repeated distraction and patient correction. However, it is always easier to make a habit than to break one.

A few pointers to good habit formation:

1. Be consistent. Do not reprove the baby for a certain action one time and ignore it the next.
2. Try to help the baby understand if he is old enough. If not, you can only rely on simple repetition.
3. Even if the baby can understand, repeat, repeat, repeat!
4. Praise accomplishment always.
5. Be patient with failure. Just persist in the effort. Do not overemphasize it.
6. Do not insist on a certain action if it is not important and the baby shows marked resistance.
7. Remain calm. Avoid a "contest" with the baby.

8. If you can get him to "want" to do it, he will, even if his motive is just to please you.

There are really two major problems involved in habit formation in babies and young children—the parent must encourage the building of good habits and also discourage the bad. Habits of deceitfulness, cheating, disobedience, saying no, hurting other children, being selfish, etc., are built by repeated practice. Habits of thoughtfulness, obedience, cooperation, friendliness and emotional control are also the result of practice. None of these habits are "bad" or "good" from the young child's viewpoint. No moral judgments are permissible where a baby is concerned. It is always the educator's responsibility. The parent's chief function in child rearing is guidance. He must show the child how—and then help him along the right road. But it is not always easy.

Don't let the baby get satisfaction from disagreeable behavior. Show disapproval, gently yet firmly, *every time* he is naughty. That does not mean bicker about unimportant trifles—but once you have decided an action merits disapproval, be consistent. It is unwise to scold a child once for throwing things and at another time ignore it. Also, it is unwise to permit him to throw a plastic cup, yet to react violently when he throws (and breaks) one of your best china teacups. The baby cannot discriminate on the basis of value. If you permit him to throw the one, he feels justified in throwing the other.

Always see that he gets satisfaction from acceptable behavior. Show him desirable ways of getting attention. Remove attention when he misbehaves. *Never threaten to withdraw love.* Love is the child's security and should not be used as a weapon. There are always other ways.

Don't make a practice of giving the baby what he cries for. If you do, he will very soon cry for whatever he wants.

Teach by example. For instance, if you always say "please" and "thank you" to him, he will learn automat-

HABITS—GOOD AND BAD

ically. Remember, he copies your responses and reactions —bad as well as good.

Don't pamper for small hurts, or he will make a great fuss over them. Be kind and gentle, but praise him for courage.

Rather than saying "don't" too often, give him something to *do*. Instead of "Don't go out in the hall", say: "Johnny's going to close the door." Let him try, then praise him. Of course, it won't always work, but it will very often avert annoying situations.

Praise is far better than punishment; whenever possible use it. Punishment should be reserved for more serious and dangerous situations.

Don't emphasize the wrong . . . always emphasize the right way. Never demonstrate an incorrect action—for example, "Don't do it this way", as that will stick with him and he may forget the "don't." Say "Keep your tongue in your mouth", rather than "Don't stick your tongue out", or, "Hold this tightly", rather than "Don't drop it".

Try to say "We don't do that", or, "Nobody does it that way". Young children like to belong to the group and be socially acceptable. Even before your baby seems old enough to participate he can already sense approval and disapproval on the part of adults.

Instead of highlighting a "disagreeable" procedure, such as going to bed, make a game of undoing buttons, pulling off clothes, having a bath, etc. If it is treated as a game he may look forward to it.

Always stress the positive.

The young child learns best by doing. Let him help to pack away his toys, hold his spoon, dress himself, even when it's more trouble that way. Let him learn to blow his nose, etc. Don't let him become too dependent. Dependence is a habit that carries through life.

Use the same words for habitual commands. "That's enough, now", when you want crying stopped, etc.

"What's the matter", when he seems distressed, etc. With all of the things he must learn, it simplifies matters greatly for him if he can recognize instructions and questions easily. New words often require much thought on his part.

Encourage, don't discourage. Parents often overlook the fact that a baby's small failures distress him. Above all he needs self-confidence, or he will become shy and cowardly.

Try to get the baby to come to you willingly after he playfully runs away. This may take some more time than simply running after him and grabbing him, but it will prevent the formation of a "running away" habit, and the constant need for chasing him. Hold out your arms and smile as though it were a game.

It is impossible to deal effectively with the subject of habit formation without discussing the problem of discipline and punishment. No matter how affectionate and willing a child may be, he cannot discriminate wisely between acceptable and unacceptable conduct, certainly not at an early age. Even when he knows what is expected of him, he will not always do it. Quite often he will seem to disobey deliberately. Whether or not this is the case, he must be corrected.

Discipline and punishment are controversial words. Many different definitions have been offered. Actually, the word "discipline" can be used to refer to milder forms of correction, "punishment" to sterner measures. No matter which word is used, the purpose of these measures should be clear. By discipline OR punishment we want to build the child's own judgment. Our aim is not to make him obey us but to teach him correct habits and to help him adjust to the outside world. If the result of any punishment is to build up a resentment in the child toward the punisher, it has failed in its purpose. The aim is to build good habits in the young child and check the unfavorable ones for his own sake, and for the sake of his family and the society in which he lives. The better his habit system is, the more favorably he will adjust and the more friendly his family and the outside world will feel toward him.

If a child gets his way by whining, crying, having tantrums and making a general nuisance of himself, it is unfortunate but true that the people who give him his way are to blame for the situation. And it is safe to assume that basically he is an unhappy child. He dominates, but he does not win, for every child yearns for love and approval. It is to help him gain this that we discipline or punish him, *not* to make him suffer for what he has done to displease.

Ideally, when the child is disciplined it should help him to understand what he has done that is wrong. Of course the younger he is the less he will understand, but even a tone of voice can convey the idea, and young children can learn to obey satisfactorily without knowing the reasons.

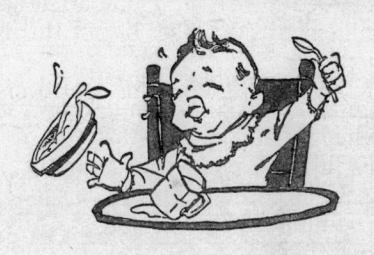

Discipline and Punishment

by **Alfred J. Vignec, M.D.**

PARENTS often come to me with questions about discipline and punishment. They worry if they do—and they worry if they don't. There is no rule for the amount of discipline or the severity of the punishment any child needs. Parental control should first of all be a matter of friendly control; and both discipline and punishment should be administered within the framework of friendliness. But there are certain facts about these two phases of child management that every parent should know before he practices either one.

Make the discipline *appropriate*. Let it come immediately. Let it take the same form for the same offense whenever possible. Have confidence in your child's desire to be good. Let him know you believe in him even when he is naughty—that you dislike what he is doing, not him. A child who feels that he is "bad" will never make an earnest effort to be good. Such a child has a poor opinion of himself and is easily tempted to do the wrong thing as a means of getting attention or expressing his resentment. Once the child gets the impression that he is strongly disapproved of, he will no longer be outgoing, friendly or cooperative. Analyze your own emotions. You don't usually strive to please those you are hostile to, but those you love and admire.

If your child knows he can count on your affection

and fairness, he will do a great deal for you, and the relationship will be a wholesome and pleasant one for both of you.

Learn to use psychology. Let the punishment fit the offense. If he kicks, take off his shoe. If he strikes with a toy, take it away. If he bites, try putting his own finger or hand into his mouth and say, "bite that."

If he is doing something that annoys you, you may want to force him to do it as a means of making him stop. One mother whose child persisted in striking matches stood by and made him strike an entire box full of kitchen matches. He never wanted to again. This, of course, might not be effective with every child, but the principle is not a bad one. If he slams the door every time he comes in, make him return to it and slam it five times, etc. In order to avoid the annoyance to himself, the child often stops the distasteful action.

Nagging, preaching or slapping indiscriminately are not effective. Spanking—a last resort.

Spanking should be used only when absolutely necessary. If the child is spanked, it must be done immediately after the offense if it is to be effective. The spanking itself should be short and not accompanied by threats—it should never be done while the adult is in a temper or has lost control of himself, because then it causes genuine fear—even panic. Remember that the adult is stronger than the child and the child knows it. Always spank with the hand—you then have a measure of how much you are hurting. Reserve spanking as a punishment for serious or dangerous situations.

The child should not be frightened as a punishment. This can only give rise to fears which it will later be your job to break down. Do not make exaggerated threats which cannot be carried out. Putting a child in the dark is never advisable. Using loss of love as a punishment is very harmful as it creates a deep insecurity in the young child and makes him anxious and fearful. He loses his basic faith in the rightness of things. Shaming should never be used except very cautiously. Certainly the child should not be disgraced in front of any group. At most, he can be made to feel that his conduct in a given situation is not acceptable to other people.

Milder methods of discipline and punishment are always preferable if they can be used effectively. Every parent can devise systems of his own. The following often prove useful:

Deprive a child of some luxury or pleasurable activity for a time (candy, television, etc.) This is often effective. If he hits someone with a toy, take it away from him and try to tell him why, even if he seems too young to understand. After a while, return the toy, but if he repeats his aggressive behavior, take it away for a much longer period.

Ignore him if he kicks, fusses, whines or behaves disagreeably. He is trying to get attention. If he does not succeed, it has positive effect, although perhaps not immediately. It takes patience to break down a bad habit.

Isolation from the group is usually the opposite of what a child wants. He may not admit it, but he yearns to return and be a part of things again. This appropriate when his group behavior has been unsatisfactory.

Distract him if you can. Diversion is very simple and useful, especially with the younger child. If his attention can be distracted, he will often forget the mischief he was engaged in.

Don't coax when he sulks. That's what he wants. There is only one remedy for a sulky child—leave him alone. That is *not* what he wants, even though it may seem to be.

Letting him take the natural consequences of his behavior is a good method. If he throws his toys away, don't pick them up unless you are definitely playing with him. Say, "There, now you've lost it." You may

DISCIPLINE AND PUNISHMENT

prefer to warn him the first time by saying, "Next time I won't get it for you", and then don't. If he refuses to take his milk or play a game, let him miss out on it. Point out to him that he's missing something, but don't make an issue of it or show that he's annoying you.

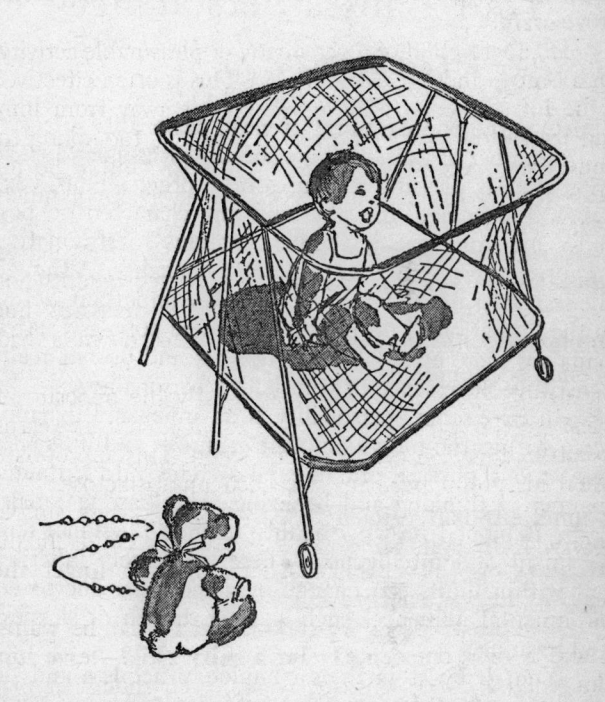

Your Baby's Personality

by **Walter J. Coville, Ph.D.**

FROM the popular point of view, personality refers to a number of traits that are socially pleasing and elicit appropriately pleasing responses from others. Thus, your baby's appearance, his physique, his characteristic postures, his smile or his unique reactions to stimulation comprise the popular concept of personality. Although the responses of others to your baby are important factors in the formation of his personality, these popularly noted traits are mere external characteristics and do not really constitute the essence of your baby's personality.

In its essence, personality is an inner and dynamic force within the individual that organizes and integrates the various physical and mental systems into a unique manner of thinking and behaving. The "raw materials" to be fashioned into personality include physique, temperament and intelligence. These are largely inherited but within limits can change over the years due to environmental influences such as food, health or sickness, and learning.

Your baby at birth is completely helpless and dependent upon others for the satisfaction of his needs and is independent only in his capacity to breathe. Strictly speaking, your baby does not as yet have a personality of his own; he has not as yet developed a characteristic manner of behaving and thinking. However, he does have the inherited "raw materials" of his potential personality and these will develop uniquely and in time within the limits set by his hereditary endowments.

The first signs of your baby's emerging personality are variously dated. For some, the first sign occurs when your baby of two weeks stops crying and stretches in a characteristic fashion toward the nipple; for others, when he stops crying upon being picked up. Some date the onset of emerging personality at 3 months when he begins to show his interest in people by a social smile, while still others at about 4 months when your baby begins to babble, eat, reach, and move about in a distinctive fashion. These characteristic traits become more conspicuous in time and at 8 months your baby makes a distinct advance in his social development. He now responds characteristically to smiling or scolding, to a friendly or angry face. He gleefully recognizes familiar people by simple hand waving but responds to strangers with caution or fear. At about 9 months, he begins to imitate simple movements. This is another important factor in the development of his personality. All this behavior, however, is sensory-motor, and your baby as yet has no concept of self.

Perhaps, a clearer emergence of your baby's personality is noted in the various manifestations of temperament. Temperament refers to one's emotional nature and more specifically to his sensitivity in responding to stimulation, his strength and speed of response, and to the quality, intensity and the various fluctuations of mood. Studies show that infants differ markedly in temperament and that, in a general way, these temperamental dispositions can be identified. Thus, one baby is sensitive, highstrung and over-active; another is unresponsive or fearful while another is stable, friendly, adaptable and not easily upset. These temperamental dispositions, however, do not predict reliably the kind of inner control your baby will have or the kind of self image that will develop in the future. Although the specific patterns of feeling, thinking and behaving in the future cannot be known in advance, the influences of environment and particularly those of significant people in the environment are extremely important in determining the development of your baby's personality.

Psychologists differ in what specific environmental factors during infancy account for the development of a stable personality. However, it is safe to conclude from their various studies that the infant in his first year of life is so plastic and resilient that no specific child training methods—such as breast feeding, gradual weaning, nursery schedules, or lack of restraint—are reliably correlated with specific personality traits that emerge later. On the other hand, their studies tend to confirm the importance of mother and the kind of "mothering" she offers her baby as a most important factor in the development of her child's personality. Specifically, this critical factor of "mothering" deals with the development of trust. Your baby is completely helpless and dependent upon others for survival. Unless he can rely upon and trust his mother his beginning in life will be very poor.

Baby's relationship with mother is his first and most meaningful experience in life. It is a critical experience because it constitutes the basis for the growth of love and trust, the taproots of his developing personality. Although your baby at birth is not yet equipped to form a personal attachment, he can feel, smell and respond to emotional warmth and acceptance and to the physical care that relieves him of pain and discomfort. This capacity for response provides the loving mother with an opportunity to nourish the taproots of his personality and form a foundation for the development of adequate personal attachments. This is accomplished by the loving mother who creates pleasant sensations by cuddling her baby warmly, holding him securely, bathing him tenderly and otherwise by caring for his needs in a fond and loving

YOUR BABY'S PERSONALITY

manner. Such care results in a pleasant relationship with mother and provides the normal baby with a basis for his own emotional security. On the other hand, the rigid, fearful or even rejecting mother, who touches or handles her baby in an anxious or hostile manner while feeding, bathing or changing him creates painful and disagreeable sensations. Later, these may be aggravated by warnings, scoldings or other punishments. Such inadequate relationships destroy trust and form the foundation for emotional insecurity and instability.

In this contact, it is also noted that some mothers may feel that problems of relationship between mother and baby are due to a clash of wills. This is not true since the infant is not equipped to do this. He is completely dependent, and his perception of the environment around him and his place in it is adequate. He just does not have the capacity to size up the situation before him and to choose to fight back. Such apparent clashes usually reflect a mother's insecurity in her relationship to the child, her own rigidity and her determination to mold her baby's behavior in accordance with a predetermined pattern. In such instances, the child is really responding to some kind of pain and discomfort rather than to a stand taken against the person caring for him.

Optimum personality development is assured if your baby experiences a continuous loving relationship. The nature of this loving relationship involves an attitude of supreme concern for the growth and happiness of your baby; an attitude of responsibility, which enables the mother to respond not only to the expressed but even to the unexpressed needs of her baby; an attitude of respect which enables the mother to view her baby objectively and to accept him as he is; and finally, an attitude of knowledge, which enables the mother to respond to the very core of her baby's being rather than to any superficial characteristic of personality. If such love and understanding is given to the baby in these early and critical years, he can be expected to mature, capable of accepting love from others and also of giving it without demanding immediate rewards in return. Thus, continuous, loving and satisfying experiences with mother provide the basis for your baby's feelings of trust, confidence and security. These then enable him to mature and continue his successful adaptation to his environment. On the other hand, if he is frustrated in satisfying his needs, anxiety develops and retards his personality growth.

Thus, your baby, nourished by the warmth and security of love continues to grow. His attachment to mother, first appearing early in life, helps him to master his infantile impulses, overcome his fear of losing mother, and gain increasing security in his dealings with the environment. Although a mother's influence upon her baby's personality is indeed critical, the infant's personality in essence is not yet formed during the first year of life. However, the foundation and the taproot of the personality is in place, and the kind of personality that eventually evolves depends upon the nature of continued early life experiences.

It is safe to say that early life experiences, rooted in loving relationships first with mother and then with other significant people in the environment, insure the development of a secure and stable personality, whereas experiences of dissatisfaction or deprivation will result in personality retardation.

The Aggressive Child

by Alfred J. Vignec, M.D.

AGGRESSIVENESS is basically a good and useful trait. If properly directed, it can give rise to leadership and general accomplishments in many fields. Yet to parents it can be a worrisome quality. Distorted, as it so often is in young children, it causes upheavals, and the truly aggressive child is seldom welcomed in a play group, or by other parents.

The aggressive child strikes out. He hits, he grabs, he argues, he fights, he stands competition poorly. Often he throws things. He may employ temper tantrums as a means to an end. He is generally loud, noisy, and may be erratic and unpredictable. He is often described as "hard to handle." As an infant, the potentially aggressive child is often a bundle of energy—kicks, squirms, does not like to be held, has what adults describe as a "will of his own."

Again, as with the timid child, innate personality is a definite factor. The mere fact that the aggressive young child was often an energetic, highly active infant indicates to the observer that there is a continuity, and that certain elements leading to aggressive later behavior were born with the baby, so to speak. The term "inherited" may be employed, but by what mysterious process this hereditary transmission takes place is far too complicated for the average parent to explore. There may be no aggressive person in the infant's immediate background, yet this tendency may be obvious and may be there from the beginning.

Again, however, the direction the innate aggressive tendency takes is strongly influenced by the surroundings and by the child's position in his family. Marked aggression with troublesome overtones can be emphasized by many factors. Over-discipline, which makes the timid child more timid, increases aggression in the child who points in this direction. He resents being handled too strictly and lashes out at his fellows to express this. Over-indulgence may also bring about aggressive behavior. The so-called "spoiled" child, lacking proper guidance and getting "his way" by yelling and shouting tends to employ the same method at play and in school because at home it has proven effective. "Sibling rivalry," the sadly overworked brother-sister competition which is blamed for so much, can also play a part here. In the oldest child, aggressive behavior can be an effect of too much authority granted this child by the parents—in the youngest, it can be caused by too much indulgence on the part of parents and older children—and in the "middle" child it can be an attention-getting device, to avoid or counteract the danger of "middle-child obscurity". He who hammers is heard. He who fights is noticed. To middle children, being noticed, for whatever cause, is often very important. In fact, most aggressive children, whatever their position in the family structure, are by nature attention-getters.

At times aggressiveness is the result of general emotional disturbance, and if this is the reason, the cause must be discovered. Parental discord, a broken home, an unsatisfactory parent-child relationship, illness on the child's part, or a general sense of inferiority may be causative factors. The child who employs aggressiveness because of genuine emotional upheaval may not be innately aggressive at all, but may be merely reacting to circumstances.

Any prolonged frustration also feeds aggression. The unsuccessful or unpopular child who finds life too much to handle often employs this weapon, usually with little or no success. His aggressiveness makes him even less acceptable, he is even more defeated, and a vicious cycle comes into being.

The aggressive child very frequently resorts to bullying, venting his spleen on smaller or weaker objects. Aggressiveness and destructiveness are often intimately related. Who or what the child attacks may be a measure of his self-confidence or lack of it. Some children attack their equals in strength, and there are even those who persistently besiege those stronger than themselves and are just as persistently defeated. These children simply refuse to acknowledge that stronger children exist—a rather interesting phenomenon, to say the least. More so because aggression of the more successful type is often intimately related to persistence. Coupled with good judgment (which develops with maturity) this is certainly a most desirable trait. The man who refuses to accept defeat despite buffetings often contributes very positively to our society. Of course, a child cannot continually come home bloodied and unbowed—the parent must introduce the factors of common sense and prudence into the child's conduct.

The parent of an aggressive child invariably has one major question—what to do about it? As with any other problem of early (and also later) childhood, it pays to devote some energy to ferreting out the cause, if this is possible. Some clue, at least, can usually be obtained. The problems of over-discipline and over-indulgence call for a change in the parents' basic handling of the child. If sibling rivalry is paramount, or if the child is reacting to his position in the family, parental interference is almost always necessary. The middle child's rights should be recognized—he should be made to feel important. The oldest child's authority may need curbing—the youngest may need to learn sharing and respect for the rights of others. If emotional disturbance is the chief factor, professional help may be needed.

In general, however, there are certain things to be kept in mind about children who express themselves by aggressive behavior. Such children very frequently—in fact, almost always—have a great need to excel. They may or may not lack confidence. But something is wrong. They are not, by their own standards at least, achieving success. The successful child does not need to be aggressive. His excellences in certain directions, his abilities, and his qualities of leadership are recognized, and he is happy and at peace. The little fighter, on the other hand, is somehow falling short. Perhaps his goals are too high. Maybe he does not have quite the ability he longs for.

Build your aggressive child's confidence. See that he excels in some field. Praise freely. If possible, help him to find a mode of self-expression. If the child leans toward collecting things, start him early. Even an eager 2-3 year old can derive great pleasure from amassing what he considers a magnificent collection of stones of various colors, shapes and sizes. Almost anything can be collected successfully, with a little guidance from Mommy and Daddy, and tremendous satisfaction can be gained by the child. He feels important. Generally relatives and friends join in the praise when they visit, and the small child literally beams when he is the center of this type of adult attention. He has actually done Something, and people notice. Sometimes aggression can be worked off by dramatic efforts (on a very simple scale, of course) or dancing, especially for girls. There are many other possibilities for providing useful activities which require effort expenditure and reap satisfaction.

Aggressive children are often potential leaders, and do not know how to go about it. Some lack popularity and this frustration makes them hate others. A child's appearance may attract or repel his playmates and adults as well. Tasteful, colorful clothing (not necessarily expensive), plus personal cleanliness and neatness are a good start for any child. The mother can help a great deal in the development of social consciousness and confidence. Small gatherings, called "parties" but kept very simple, in which the small "host" or "hostess" is allowed to participate, helping to serve juice or cookies, planning the games with Mommy, etc., are very helpful to eager frustrated little ones. Just a warm welcome to playmates makes them want to come. When the child is overbossy, he drives others away. This should be tactfully pointed out to him by Mommy and Daddy.

Many of these children are basically dynamic, want success, want to be first, or they will not compete. Often they lack the innate ability to be first, and they wage a constant war with the destiny that gave others a better natural endowment. These youngsters must first of all be understood and accepted for what they are and exactly as they are. It is quite understandable that Johnny may feel he must be at the head of the class or first in all sports if these are his parents' spoken or unspoken standards. If the parent accepts the aggressive child's limitations, even at an early age, he too in time will learn to respect himself for what he actually is and perform to the best of his own ability.

Try to instill a sense of sportsmanship into your little fighter. Teach him to protect those younger and weaker than himself. At least then his bloody nose will be in a good cause. Many aggressive children desperately want a cause as an outlet for their instincts and energies, and are avid in its defense when they have it. They fall readily into the spirit of the crusader, sometimes at a surprising early age. There are some children who cannot be passive—they must be colorful, active, alive at every moment. They are bursting with energy which, if misdirected, can certainly be trying. They are at their best when busy.

Occasionally, however, it is not the outgoing, active child, but the silent one who is aggressive and even hostile to his environment. This problem is generally harder to handle. This child's frustration often lies deeper; he may have masked it even from himself. He is taking his spite out on his environment, and may even be compensating for timidity. If his problems can be drawn out into the open and his conflicts solved, his aggression may disappear entirely.

Reasoning with the child and discussing his problems in a friendly fashion when he is old enough to understand (simple language and terms for young children, of course) is a good attempt. It does not always bear fruit, however. Some children do not respond to this effort at all. Others take an interest, even at an early age, and benefit in greater or lesser measure.

The parents of an innately aggressive child will never have a dull home; this much at least is fairly certain. But many exciting and interesting experiences can be shared. This type of child is a challenger. If the challenge is met, much may be accomplished.

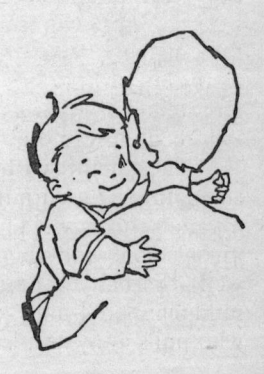

The Timid Child

by **Alfred J. Vignec, M.D.**

TIMIDITY or "shyness" appears even in infancy. Everyone has come across the baby who cannot be approached by strangers, cries readily, clings to his parents, and does not seem quite able or ready to face his small world. Equally familiar is the toddler who wails and hides when guests appear and is assailed by manifold fears and night terrors—the preschool child who sulks or retreats or sticks his tongue out at an unfamiliar face even though it is smiling—the kindergartner who becomes sick with fear when he must "leave home" for the first time and go to school.

At least an element of this "timidity" is usually inborn, although very adverse circumstances and surroundings can break the spirit of almost any child. But the fact remains that many infants are spontaneously outgoing from the cradle, while others have a more reserved nature and tend to withdraw from strangers and unfamiliar objects almost at the dawn of awareness.

The infant with a wary approach is particularly susceptible to environmental distortion, and may react in a variety of ways. The most obvious is the quiet, submissive role, and this is the most socially acceptable as well—the baby or small child is merely shy, dependent, mild-mannered and gentle. Less acceptable is the child who pulls away and is timid about things or people, submissive away from home and demanding and tyrannical with his parents. Most objectionable of all is the child who is sulky or even hostile to cover his timidity—who appears superior, indifferent, or utterly self-contained, while he is actually the victim of loneliness, isolation and unhappiness which he shares with none. Whatever the particular expression of timidity, the child who feels inadequate is in an unenviable position—whether his unhappiness is shared or hidden, it is there and when the people whom he knows and loves let him down—as they invariably must—he feels alone in an alien world.

The most common cause of timidity is overprotection. An excessively cushioned atmosphere in the home makes the child inadequate to cope with the outside world. At home he is "understood", condoned, catered to and regarded as very important—outside he is just one of the crowd, and is expected to perform beyond his real or imagined capabilities. He has been dressed, he can't tie his own shoes when the others can, and so on. Criticism breaks him down, and he reacts with tears. When he cannot get what he wants he also cries. He is often considered babyish by his fellows, yet they frequently give in to him, especially in the younger years, rather than cause a scene and hubbub which will disrupt their play. Even his parents often desert him. The overprotective parent first causes the problem, then resents the child for his poor performance and rejects and scolds him for it. This only brings about a state of greater confusion and the child's adjustment patterns become even less satisfactory.

In contrast, the too strictly handled child also often feels insecure; perhaps because of undue criticism or excessive severity, he has come to feel inadequate and reacts with one or the other type of withdrawal. This child is seldom the tyrant in the home, and some of his older reactions may differ as well, but he is also afraid of the unknown and the unfamiliar and tends to be shy and unventuresome.

It is not always easy to correct the difficulty even when the parent is aware of the cause. Emotions play a large role, and the emotional patterns which caused the parent to overprotect or overdiscipline in the first place are probably still present. Parental self-discipline is, as usual, the first step toward correcting the difficulties of the child.

The timid infant should be greatly encouraged whenever possible to go to strangers and to dare. He will require more comforting and reassuring than the infant of the same age who has a naturally outgoing and venturesome disposition. A timid baby cannot just be handed to strangers and permitted to cope with his panic. Neither can a small child overcome his fears and shyness merely because he is pressured to do so.

First, he must be made to feel as secure as possible in his environment, inside of the home and out. This means he must be permitted to do what the others in his age group are doing. He cannot be wrapped in cotton wool—excuses should not be made for him by a zealous mother who stands as a shield between him and his world. On the other hand, neither should he be criticized for his imperfections to such an extent that his self-confidence is impaired.

His parents should teach him so that he is able to compete and feel self-assurance. Yet they must especially let the timidly-inclined child feel that they are always there to help and guide when needed. The amount of help must be rationed to the child who has been helped too much in the past, but this should be done kindly and firmly. The child who has been handled too strictly should be praised—in fact, praise for honest accomplishment is good medicine for any child.

Above all, taunting by parents about shyness or timidity is unforgivable. The child often hates this trait in himself and would give a great deal to be able to overcome it.

Whenever possible, people from outside the family group should enter the timid child's environment. Playmates are of primary importance. If there are children in the neighborhood, the mother should invite them in, to play or even in for simple lunches. It may be some time before the child who clings to home and mother will consent to visit in other children's homes alone, but after a while his tight wall of reserve may crack and he may begin to expand his field of interest and endeavor. It is also helpful to take him for visits to other people's homes, when the mother or another familiar adult is present.

If there are no other children in the neighborhood and if it is financially feasible, nursery school is sometimes helpful to the timid child. However, it is not a universal prescription, and if strong persuasion must be employed to pry the young child loose from his home and mother, failure is more frequent than success. Nursery school is practical only if the child is ready for it. Otherwise, he may fight it by one method or another—by night terrors, nausea, vomiting, crying spells, etc.—until he is of necessity withdrawn from the threatening situation. If this occurs, he may build up harmful prejudices against school in general, which gives rise to more distressing problems in the future.

Whether or not the child can cope with nursery school, the mother should take him out into the world of strangers whenever possible, and quiet his fears and misgivings with patience and understanding. Even the supermarket is filled with possibilities. He can collect small items, take vegetables to be weighed (alone, if possible, with the mother unobtrusively alert in the background,) and help to unload at the checkout.

He should be praised and even occasionally rewarded for acts which require daring on his part, even though the spontaneously outgoing child may do the same things without effort or need of commendation. The world is not the same place to all children—what is a stellar accomplishment for one may be commonplace or even boring to another.

The mother of a timid child should ask herself whether or not she is clinging to him too much because of some emotional need of her own, thus in turn giving rise in him to an excessive dependence on her.

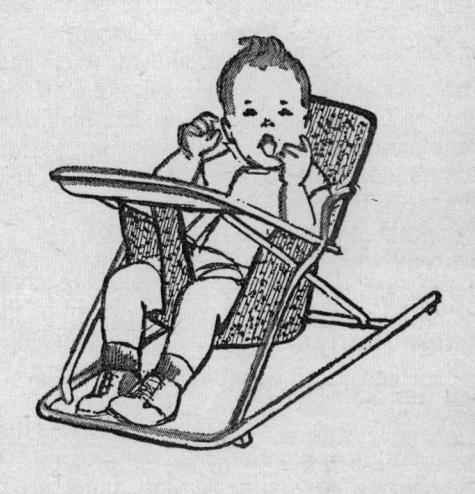

Stuttering

by Jacques P. Penn, Ph.D.

DOES your 2, 3, or 4 year old child repeat, hesitate, even block when he talks? Very probably. Does this mean he is a stutterer? Very probably not.

Why do some children become stutterers and some not? A number of theories have been offered throughout the centuries. Current thinking suspects that there may be a combination of factors that conspire to form the stuttering phenomenon. There are remarkably few physical differences between the stuttering group and the normally speaking group. Research reveals that physical movements of lips, tongue, jaw, vocal cords and lungs are quite normal among stutterers. The acts of blowing, chewing, biting, swallowing, sucking, laughing, are easily accomplished. Yet they employ the same muscle movements as the act of talking. The overwhelming majority of professional workers in the speech field look toward the environment, the emotions, the psychology of the stutterer, as the prime area of causation.

A famous study of the speech at play of a large group of normal children aged 2 to 5 revealed that there were 45 hesitations, repetitions or blocks per each 1000 sounds attempted by the children. It is generally agreed that such non-fluencies are normal expectations of speech development in young children. There is strong opinion among therapists that a stutter is "created" from this normal process by some important authority figure (mother, father, grandma, grandpa, or even lesser stars in the child's surrounding constellation of adult power) labelling the child's innocent stumbling efforts as stuttering. This word-stamp of disapproval often has attached to it stern admonitions of "speak slower" or "take a deep breath" or some similar command. Unhappy, unpleasant expressions cross the faces of loved ones. The atmosphere becomes choked with tense radiations tying up the small child's natural speaking procedure into tight little knots. The seeds of self-consciousness, apprehension and anxiety are planted in the speaking situation and stuttering is often the result.

We all have different tolerance levels for stresses and strains. Some young childrens' emerging delicate speech techniques are threatened by various environmental factors. Let us examine some of them.

Poor physical hygiene. Insufficient or improper food and sleep habits.

An overhectic program of activities. Evaluate, de-intensify or eliminate. Encourage brief rest and relaxation periods.

Disordered, chaotic family organization. Is there overly-much competition, even animosity among family members? Is it a struggle to "get the floor" in family talk around the dinner table? Structure the situation so that the weaker ones, certainly any hesitating ones, get a chance. Are other children in the immediate family clearly favored? Whose inner fibre would not be lacerated by such a covert form of rejection? Are not all of us saying in one way or another, "Tell me I exist. Acknowledge my value. Let me know."

Absent family figures. Death, divorce, separation imbalance the family structure. Working mothers, casual maids create too cool, too restrained a home atmosphere. Many young children must have frequent and strong physical demonstrations of love and affection. The need for touch and holding can become a gnawing thing.

Unrealistic family standards. Some parents have a preconceived notion of what they would like their children to be and press automatically for that image. Children must be accepted at their very own potential—not a mirage that may prove insidiously crushing in its impossible challenge. Many studies in the field indicate mothers of stutterers may often be rigid, high-strung, perfectionists, "self-sacrificing" persons.

"Momism". The hovering overprotective, shielding mother becomes oppressive. The young innocent reacts with guilt to his oppression. Caught between his desire to say, "Let me alone!" and the remorse and guilt of such socially unacceptable sentiments towards one's mother, the young speaker may acquire speech uneasiness and blocks from such ambivalence of feeling.

Inconsistent discipline. The child may feel lost and speak with lack of stability if the home does not reveal guideposts for behavior. There should be an unanimity and continuity of policy from the Executive Board (Ma and Pa) about what may or may not be permitted. Disagreement between parents about the child should be adjudicated in private caucus. Final decisions must be clearly stated and understood by the child and adhered to firmly by mother and father.

Shift of handedness. It is held by many therapists that ambidexterity may be neurologically related to poor speech maturation. The child should be encouraged, guided—but not forced—to develop and use his natural hand, right or left. This is the hand that he eats with, points with, throws with, draws and colors with, hammers with, etc. Stuttering resulting from hand-shifting practices appears to be related not to the left-right or vice-versa move, but from the pressures, tensions and general emotional distress frequently associated with the changeover.

The above mismanagements of the environment imply their own obvious and necessary changes. There is general concurrence among speech people that the healthiest prop for good, normal speech development is a happy home providing love and reliability—a secure, warm island in a bewildering world.

Proper environmental management will usually prevent the development of stuttering—and, in many cases, the early application of environmental changes will diminish or eradicate unusual manifestations of hesitations, repetitions and blocks in the young child. However, along with these attitudinal considerations or adjustments, some technical speech items may be introduced therapeutically. Providing speech victories is a helpful device that will engender feelings and memories of successes connected with speech. Such victories (none or very few hesitations, repetitions or blocks) can almost always be accomplished by any "stutterer" in talking to infants, pets, to himself aloud, by singing, talking in unison with another person, talking against great "making" noise so that he cannot hear his own voice, memorizing rhymes, dramatic parts, puppet work and other techniques not carrying the mandate of the communication of original thought to a challenging human personality.

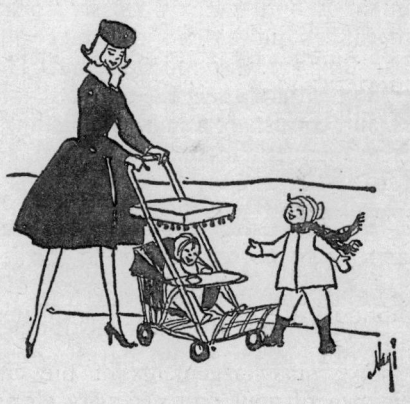

Fears In Childhood

by **Alfred J. Vignec, M.D.**

FEAR is a wholesome emotion; one which has a definite protective function in our existence and in fact, often keeps us aware. Picture a man, or even a child, without fear, striding head-on into the path of oncoming traffic, blind to the hazards of fire and water, oblivious to countless threats which life in the modern world presents daily. It is difficult to imagine such an individual remaining alive for a single day. On the other hand, uncontrolled fear is often at the root of neurosis, and even on a smaller scale, is the cause of much discomfort and difficulty in adjusting to life.

The infant is born with two basic fears; he reacts violently to sudden movements that make him feel as though he is falling, and also to loud sounds. His response to both of these situations is the same. It is called the Moro reflex, and consists of a sudden stiffening extension of the arms and legs, a clutching movement, and clenching of the fists. At the same time he quivers. This is a primitive pattern, and will appear even in very small infants.

While the infant is still quite young, he will give evidence of other and more complex fears which have apparently come to him from his environment. These may have an obvious cause, or may be mysterious in origin. They may be major or trivial.

FEARS IN CHILDHOOD

Of course, major shocks and accidents are obvious causes for future fear, and are easily traced. The child who has almost drowned shuns the water. Also, the child who has witnessed or been a party to an accident in which he or others suffered injury is likely to retain an emotional scar. These fears should be handled with patience and tolerance, and the child should be constantly reassured in the hope that his confidence will be restored.

Most fears are born because of an unhappy experience, but often it is not a particularly dramatic one, nor even dangerous. What seems fearsome and startling to the child may seem trivial and inconsequential to the adult.

It is because of this difference in evaluating a situation that a parent often has difficulty in determining the origin of a child's troublesome fear, although he himself was actually present at its inception. Then, too, a situation or circumstance may bother one child in a group, while none of the others present react at all. For example, one little girl of two was so terrified because a squirrel jumped on her hand while she was feeding it a nut that her whole attitude toward animals changed. She feared them all. Her mother was quite puzzled by this because the other children were delighted and thrilled with the feel of the squirrel's tiny claws on their hands.

Some children are unquestionably more inclined to be fearful than others. Parents describe them variously as "high strung," "nervous," "tense," etc. Whatever the terminology may be, they do need extra consideration, encouragement, security and confidence.

Children acquire many of their fears by "contagion" from an adult, usually the mother. The child whose mother fears lightning will tremble with her during a storm, often even hiding when it thunders. The small and inconsequential fears of parents are also transmitted, often unconsciously. A fearful parent who expresses her anxieties freely often creates a deep insecurity in the child.

This is the type of child who comes to feel that everything strange or difficult poses a threat, and he is hounded into flight by situations which most children meet with equanimity. If a parent is fearful or apprehensive, she (or he) should make every effort to protect the child from becoming a party to these doubts and uncertainties.

Some fears seem to arise from nowhere. Many a mother points with confusion to one child in her brood who fears dogs or water. Strive as she will, she cannot explain or understand it. "None of the others are that way. Nothing ever happened to him. He's always been afraid." This sort of situation is apparent in institutional children, who often react negatively to their first exposure to some object or situation which is not ordinarily frightening.

One little girl of one-and-a-half who had never before seen a live animal, reacted with such dread that she could not bear to approach (or see anyone else approach) a bird. Others react to water in much the same manner. Actually, when the origin of a fear is obscure, it is just as well to accept and deal with it without attempting to understand it.

There are several questions the mother should ask herself before attempting to cope with fear in her child.

First, is the fear justified? Even if it is disproportionate, a fear of water, for example, has a very sound basis as water can kill. Some children fear fire—even fear the flare of a match or the light of a candle.

Is the fear drastic enough to merit attention, or is it trivial enough to be ignored? One criterion here is the amount of discomfort the fear is causing the child. Any fear, however unimportant it may seem, deserves attention if the child suffers as a result of it. Some fears are transient. Fear of the dark, for example, often disappears as the child familiarizes himself with day and night. In other words, he "outgrows" it as he grows up.

Overcoming a troublesome fear gives the child tremendous confidence in himself; gives the parent a sense of accomplishment and triumph; and strengthens the parent-child relationship.

Fears must be handled carefully if any success is to be attained. The small child is usually aware that his fear is exaggerated—he already feels different from others because of it—and is usually sensitive as a result.

He will react poorly to being told "Now don't be silly; it's nothing. Nobody else is afraid." Anything that sounds even remotely like scolding or censure will meet with further resistance. Force will only intensify and strengthen the fear. He wants to be respected as an individual—to be accepted and understood. You and he are allies, to make him less afraid.

Unconditioning of fears can be begun at an early age. The one-and-a-half-year-old already mentioned, who could not even endure seeing a loved adult approach a sparrow, eventually gained enough confidence at two years of age to pet a horse. The process of learning was fun although there were a few ticklish moments.

First, the adult went close to the birds in the child's presence (though it caused her to cry)—speaking gently to her and reassuring her that there was nothing to fear. This was repeated until she no longer cried.

Then the adult approached larger animals in turn—pigeons, kittens, cats, then dogs—always reassuring, never coaxing the child to join her, or mentioning fear. At last the child no longer cried when the adult approached or petted animals. She was sure now, at least, of the other's confidence and complete safety.

The next step was for her to hold the hand of the adult and walk toward sparrows and pigeons together—later the larger animals in turn—always being reassured, nexer coaxed or forced. In time, she timidly fed and even touched them. These triumphs evoked squeals of mingled awe and delight. She could scarcely believe she was so brave!

It sounds simple, but was not, always. The process took six months or more, and there were many days when the little one retreated, and was allowed to retreat, and nothing was accomplished. There were also days when there were tears, and then for a while no efforts were made at all.

Lack of force is the most important factor. Gentle encouragement and a touch of persuasion are acceptable, but force only gives rise to resistance, resentment, and even fear of the person who is forcing. Disapproval on the part of the parent makes the child feel small, hate himself for his fear, and react poorly to the parents' role as well. Patience, tolerance and understanding are the best weapons. The child does not want to be afraid. He wants to feel brave and strong.

If the child is in general "anxious" with many unfounded fears, it would be wise for the mother to make sure that he is secure and happy, and that the competitive situations in his life are not too much for him. Some children who seem to fear things and situations are suffering from a genuine sense of inadequacy, and this should be looked into.

Wholesome fear of genuine dangers should be guided into the proper channels, so that the child develops caution and judgment. "Accident-prone" children are often children "without fear," and these, ironically enough, must be "taught to fear" until a proper sense of danger is achieved. Do not be deceived, however. The accident-prone child is, as a rule, a basically insecure child.

SECTION VI

Special Health Review

Health Record

by R. Cannon Eley, M.D.

Use this page to keep an accurate medical record of your baby's progress. You will find this information invaluable in future years. It will provide facts about your child's medical history for school applications, for military and employment records, for doctors who may need them.

	Doctor	Dates
Chicken Pox		
Regular Measles		
German Measles		
Mumps		
Whooping Cough		
Scarlet Fever		
Roseola		
Tonsillitis		
Tonsillectomy		
or Adenoidectomy		
Bronchitis		
Pneumonia		
Poliomyelitis		

Influenza ....

Allergies   To Drugs ....
  Animals .... Pollens ....
  Foods .... Clothing ....
Rheumatic Fever ....
or Arthritis ....
Convulsions ....
Ear Disturbances ....
Fractures ....
Operations ....
Blood Type ....

IMMUNIZATIONS   First   Boosters

Smallpox ....

Diphtheria—Tetanus—
Whooping Cough—Polio
(Course Consists of 3 Injections) ....

Poliomyelitis Vaccine—
Sabin *(3 Swallows)* ....

Poliomyelitis Vaccine—
Salk *(4 Injections)* ....

Measles Vaccine *(One Dose)* ....

Mumps Vaccine ....

Tuberculin Test ....

PKU Test ....

Health Tips

by R. Cannon Eley, M.D.

THE first year of a baby's life is a time of worry for his parents. Fortunately, most of this worry is unnecessary. Baby's illnesses during that first year fall into familiar patterns, most of which are routine, quickly-cured ailments. Here is a manual of good health tips.

COLIC: A disturbance which is common during the baby's first three months. It is characterized by painful crying, distressing to the mother, and by what appears to be an insatiable appetite. The baby's abdomen becomes hard and distended due to air collecting in the loop of the bowel. As a rule, the cause is improper feeding, although occasionally, it may be caused by bacterial action within the bowel, allergy or hunger. The baby will cry at regular intervals; and will seem to be in great pain. Try placing him face down across your knees and rubbing his back. A warm tub bath sometimes help. If the condition persists, check with your doctor.

CROUP: Inflammatory conditions of the larynx and vocal cords will often produce what is commonly called "croup." Croup causes swelling of the tissues and the closing of the air passages. When this occurs there is difficulty in breathing and a characteristic "brassy" cough. Croup may be mild or severe; but most babies respond to such treatment as the steam tent, the inhalation of oxygen, and the use of special antibiotics, which forestall and prevent attacks as well as relieving them.

COLDS: Or as they should be called, "respiratory infections" are the mysteries of modern medicine. Some colds are caused by viruses; others by bacterial infections; still, others are identified as allergies. Young babies are especially susceptible to cold infections. No specific cure has been found for colds; with babies, bed rest, fluids, drugs to reduce temperature are the best treatments. As the baby becomes older and has repeated colds, he may gradually develop his own immunity.

EAR ACHE: Ear infections in babies and young children are extremely painful; fortunately antibiotics help control these infections. When the eardrum becomes inflamed, the baby will become irritable, fretful and feverish —will cry out in pain—and usually put his hand to his affected ear. The ear may look red; sometimes there will be discharge from it. It is most important to see the doctor when the baby develops earache.

CONSTIPATION: The idea that a baby must have one or more stools a day to be well is no longer tenable. Occasionally a baby eating solid foods will have two or three bowel movements a day; another baby will have only one movement a day, or one every two days. This isn't necessarily abnormal unless it indicates a change from an established pattern. Each baby has an individual nervous system and the bowel has a tendency to regulate its own performance. Formula-fed infants can usually be relieved of constipation by increasing the amount of sugar in their diets and perhaps reducing the total intake of milk. The use of enemas, lubricants, laxatives, etc. is not encouraged except in cases where the stool has become hard, dry, lumpy and cannot be expelled. Then consult the doctor about what to do.

DIARRHEA: This is the term used to describe frequent fluid bowel passages of varying odor and color. Diarrhea is rarely related to food intake, especially with infants. It is more often caused by infection in the bowel or elsewhere in the body. Persistent diarrhea should be promptly reported to your physician. He may prescribe a special diet and medication. Small amounts of boiled water or broth may be given safely until the doctor has ordered more specific remedies.

VOMITING: There is a difference between vomiting and "spitting up." The latter is usually associated with a feeding and is nothing to worry about. It usually consists of a mouthful of milk, curdled in appearance, which the baby brings up and dribbles on its chin. Sometimes a baby lying face down in his crib will bring up small quantities of milk; even this is no cause for alarm. Vomiting on the other hand, can be caused by an infection, or a stomach irritation from something in the food. Unless there is a physical defect such as pylorospasm or pyloric stenosis, marked by vomiting with great force, ordinary vomiting will pose no special problem to your doctor.

FEVER: Fever often accompanies a cold but in young or very ill infants, fever is an unreliable sign. High fevers tend to occur in the early months and become less common as the child grows older. Aspirin may safely be given in a dosage of one grain per year of age up to ten years. Sponging the body with tepid water will help lower the temperature temporarily and will comfort the baby. Your physician should be consulted immediately.

ALLERGIES: Allergies are sensitivities to certain substances, such as foods, pollen, weeds, feathers, animal dander, etc., which cause a reaction when encountered. Allergy symptoms vary from runny nose, coughing, heavy breathing, wheezing and cramps to actual vomiting and skin eruptions. When these signs are seen, they may not necessarily be of an allergic nature. Nevertheless, if they persist, it is a good plan for the mother to make a list of the potential irritants the baby has been exposed to over a two-day period just prior to an attack of sneezing, coughing, diarrhea or other symptom of allergy. It may not be needed, but it will be helpful to the doctor in making his diagnosis.

SKIN IRRITATIONS: After digestive problems, skin irritations are perhaps the most common first-year complaints of new mothers. *Diaper rash*, most common of these, is easily preventable by cleanliness both in washing and changing the baby's diapers. The use of a good baby product that is a diaper-rash preventive is recommended after each diaper change. *Thrush monilia* are red elevated spots. It may grow in the diaper area or in the skin under the neck where it is warm and moist. It frequently occurs after diarrhea. It may also appear as a white, caked layer on the tongue, lips and gums. It should be treated by the doctor. *Cradle cap*, another type of rash, is thought to be an allergic condition. Treat it by loosening the crust on the scalp with warm oil, followed by a shampoo and scraping the scales from the scalp with a fine tooth comb. *Prickly heat* is usually the result of overdressing the baby. Liberal application to the body of a good absorbent baby powder is the best remedy for the condition, as well as dressing baby in lighter, more absorbent clothing.

FRESH AIR: Just when the baby can go outside depends on the area in which you live. It is generally felt that a baby may safely be put outside at about two months of age as long as he is in a protected area, warm, comfortable and the temperature is not below freezing. The time should be short at first (20 to 30 minutes) and gradually increased to several hours. He will probably be just as well and healthy inside the house near an open window. Sun baths in the summer are not recommended by some physicians who feel that the actual act of sun bathing is unnecessary if a child is outdoors in his ordinary daily routine. Vitamin D is absorbed through the skin in this way just as through actual sun bathing sessions—and the browner a baby gets, the less ultraviolet ray his skin absorbs.

BRUISES: Apply cold compresses to injured part for half hour (no ice next to skin). If skin is broken, treat as a cut. For serious injuries always consult your physician without delay.

CUTS: Small. Wash with clean water and soap. Hold under running water. Apply sterile gauze dressing. Large— Apply dressing. Press firmly to stop bleeding—use tourniquet only if necessary. Bandage. Do not use iodine or other antiseptics before the physician arrives.

BURNS: Of Limited Extent. If caused by heat, cover with gauze and bandage lightly. If caused by chemicals: Wash burned area thoroughly with water. Extensive Burns—Keep patient in flat position. Remove clothing from burned area—if it adheres to burns, leave alone. Cover with clean cloth and keep patient warm. Take patient to hospital or to a physician at once. Do not use ointments, greases, etc. Electric burns may require artificial respiration.

NOSEBLEEDS: Keep patient in sitting position; have him blow out from nose all clot and blood. Insert a wedge of cotton moistened with any of the regulation nose drops and with the finger against the outside of that nostril apply firm pressure for five minutes. If bleeding stops leave packing in place. If bleeding persists, secure medical advice.

WARTS: A wart is a harmless skin growth caused by a virus. Why some individuals are susceptible to this virus is not known. Warts are most commonly seen in children and young adults. The most frequent area is on the fingers or the back of the hands. Warts may also occur on the face and, not uncommonly, on the sole of the foot where they tend to be pushed into the skin and therefore do not protrude above the surface. These are known as plantar warts.

UMBILICAL CORD: (Navel). The navel is the cord through which nourishment is supplied to the fetus. The cord, containing a vein and two umbilical arteries, does not bleed. After the baby is born, it is permitted to dry; whereupon it falls off.

MULTIPLE BIRTHS: Twins occur approximately once in ninety births, triplets once in almost 1,000 pregnancies, quadruplets once in almost 5,000 pregnancies, and quintuplets approximately once in millions of deliveries. The peak incidence for twins occurs in women between 35 and 40, is more common in women with previous pregnancies, more common in Negroes than in Caucasians, and is least common among the Japanese.

TONSILS: The tonsils consist of lymphoid tissue located on each side of the back of the throat. Tonsils (and the adenoids which are located near them) are frequently the source of chronic and recurrent upper respiratory infections in children. Frequently the infection extends into the ear.

There is often fever which can go as high as 104°, sore throat, inability to swallow, lack of appetite, nasal obstruction, and possibly impaired hearing.

Many mild cases of tonsillitis will clear up without the use of antibiotics. Aspirin may be helpful in reducing the pain and fever. However, many cases require the use of antibiotics. Most cases clear up within seven to ten days. In severe cases tonsillectomy may be required.

TOILET TRAINING: Successful toilet training is a

complex procedure for the young child. All normal children accomplish toilet training eventually, and it is therefore simply a matter of time before the process is completely mastered. It is wise to be patient and wait until the child is sufficiently mature to master this procedure.

ACCIDENT PREVENTION: Infancy and childhood are periods in which physical abilities outstrip understanding and caution. Inevitably they are periods of accidents—some trivial, some quite serious. Every mother must act as a safety engineer, and face all of the accident possibilities, however unpleasant they may be.

These are some of the guidelines which will enable parents to protect their children: (1) Never leave a small child unattended in the home. (2) Close all doors leading to basement stairs. Insert gates at the heads of stairs. Put window guards on the windows. These measures will cut down on serious falls in the younger age groups. (3) Keep medicines in a locked medicine chest; if the medicine chest cannot be locked, find some other place for drugs. (A sliding bolt on the bathroom door that can be reached only by the adults may be a useful solution to the bathroom threat.) (4) Never take or dispense a medicine in the dark, or without checking the label and the appearance of the medication itself. (5) Make sure that bleaches, polishes, detergents, bowl cleaners, perfumes, and pesticides, etc. are inaccessible to young children. (6) Never store cleaning agents, turpentine, paint remover, or other chemicals in soda or milk bottles, nor keep them on shelves with foods.

BABY SITTERS: There are about a million persons who baby sit in the United States. Most baby sitters are teenagers, and fortunately they usually like youngsters. But the parent must remember that a baby sitter is not the parent, and therefore there are limits that must be set for the sitter. Baby sitters should not be asked to perform the functions of a trained nurse.

A baby sitter should be given an orientation talk which will include information about what the child likes, how the home is run, situations the baby sitter is to be particularly alerted to, especially those that are likely to result in accidents. Of course, the most important lesson you must get across to the baby sitter is that his or her main job is to watch the child, so that you will find him safe when you return home.

BITES, ANIMAL: Most animal bites present no special problems of infection. The risk of infection is cut further if you permit some bleeding from the wound or even encourage bleeding with slight pressure, as in the case of puncture wounds produced by a cat scratch. Wash the wound with soap and water, which may be all the first-aid procedures that are needed. If there is free bleeding, such as may occur from a dog-inflicted laceration, a clean compress can be applied and firm pressure maintained. If the skin is not penetrated by a bite, there need be no further concern. If the skin is penetrated, see your doctor. Further treatment may be necessary.

BITES, INSECT: Bites of mosquitoes and gnats will produce immediate itching, which may recur thereafter for one or more days. Such bites are generally disregarded. However, a paste of soda bicarbonate or a piece of cotton dipped in household ammonia diluted with three parts of water may be dabbed on the bite. Calamine lotion may be applied for recurrent itching.

Bee bites can be treated by removal of the stinger with a tweezer, followed by an application of ice, then by calamine lotion or a paste of bicarbonate of soda. Bee bites can be dangerous and even fatal to sensitive individuals. Indications of such sensitivity are usually local swelling, and marked general reactions such as weakness, faintness or collapse. If any such unusual reactions do occur, hypersensitivity exists.

BLEEDING: Bleeding from a large cut can be heavy if one of the larger veins or arteries is cut. The best method for control of such bleeding is to exert firm pressure, using a cloth compress on the area. In an emergency use a wad of facial tissue, a handkerchief, towel, shirt, or a pillowcase to make the compress. Press it against the bleeding area, and if the cut is on a leg or arm, elevate it to diminish bleeding. Maintain pressure for five to ten minutes, then lift part of the compress to judge whether the bleeding has come under control. If it has not, pressure can be maintained for a longer period, or even indefinitely, if necessary.

CONVULSIONS: Convulsions, often called "fits" or seizures, are caused by many different conditions. The eyes roll up into the head, the jaws are clamped shut, and the child loses consciousness as the body stiffens. Parts of the body then shake with twitching or convulsive movements. There may be difficulty in breathing, and the color of the skin may change to bluish or reddish purple. There may be some frothing at the mouth. Sometimes high fever or the onset of an illness may cause a convulsion. More serious causes of convulsions in children are brain disorders (epilepsy, brain tumors) and poisoning. Most convulsions are self-limited: the child may be unconscious for one or two minutes, then come around. Your doctor should be consulted.

ANTIBIOTICS: An antibiotic is a substance secreted by one organism which will kill other organisms—specifically bacteria and fungi. The first and best known of the antibiotics is penicillin. Its successors include sulfa drugs, streptomycin, tetracycline, and terramycin. Less well known are mycostatin, griseofulvin, kanamycin, and others which have limited but useful special application.

Recently, chemically modified forms of the naturally-occurring penicillin have appeared; these have useful new properties, including the ability to attack certain penicillin-resistant organisms.

GENES: Genes are units of heredity. They can be looked upon as a long list of controls which determine the structure and much of the functioning of offspring. The enormous number of genes present in each of us is indicated in the innumerable characteristics that are unique to one individual as compared to another: height, weight, eyes, skin and hair color, nose size, jaw formation, body build, hair distribution, intelligence (I.Q.), and musical and mathematical abilities—not to mention all of the disorders or illnesses that have a family background, such as high blood pressure, diabetes, high blood cholesterol, gout, etc.

CIRCUMCISION: Circumcision consists of surgical removal of some of the foreskin—the excess skin which conceals the head of the penis. Sometimes the foreskin is tight so that it may be difficult to pull it back. Irritation of the penis then occurs because of retained secretions (known as smegma) or even from the accumulation of small amounts of urine in this location. Circumcision performed as a religious ceremony has been practiced by the Jews and Moslems for centuries. The operation has become increasingly popular with other ethnic groups.

HEARTBURN: Heartburn refers to a burning sensation high in the upper central abdomen. It is experienced by many people after spicy, rich, greasy, or fried foods, or after they have taken too much coffee or alcohol. It is a common complaint during pregnancy, when it is caused by various functional changes in the behavior of the digestive tract. Heartburn is probably not due to "excess acidity," but neutralizing stomach acids will help heartburn as well as other digestive complaints.

HEMORRHOIDS: Hemorrhoids are small distended veins in the region of the anus or rectal opening. Those just inside the opening are covered by the lining of the anus and are called internal hemorrhoids; those exterior to this are covered by skin and are called external hemorrhoids. Anything that raises the pressure within the veins of the rectal region may bring on or aggravate hemorrhoids. Pregnancy is one of the most common aggravating factors, as is also chronic constipation and straining at stool.

SICK CHILD: Sick children usually have no appetite for solid foods. The best thing to do is to nourish them with fruit or fruit juices; liquids, such as bouillon; weak tea; clear soup; sodas, milk, and ice cream. Mashed banana may be given in orange juice, or other fresh fruit mashed in fruit juice. This provides glucose (sugar) and some fluid. Other foods which are both nutritious and easy to digest are Jello, custard, rice pudding, mashed potatoes, or any easy-to-swallow food. If a child vomits there is medicine which can be given to stop the vomiting. Consult your doctor.

IMMUNIZATIONS: There are many diseases today which your child will never contract if he is immunized against them. In previous years thousands of children died during epidemics of diseases which can now be prevented. It is, therefore, important and necessary for you to give your child all the injections which have been developed to protect him. Epidemics still do occur, but if this happens your child will be protected. Get in touch with your physician to arrange for this protection.

INTUSSUSCEPTION: This is a form of intestinal obstruction which occurs mostly in young male children.

A portion of the lower intestine turns inside itself and blocks the passage of food. This causes severe colicky pain, fever, and strangely-colored bowel movements because of some passage of blood in the stools. A sausage-shaped mass may sometimes be felt in the abdomen. This condition requires immediate medical attention.

SPEECH: All early sounds in infancy are impulsive and aimless. By two months of age they have generally become cooing and gurgling sounds; at four months there are consonants followed by vowels; at eight months, certain syllables and then "Mama" and "Dada." At eighteen months, words may be accompanied by movements and gestures. At twenty-four months, short sentences of three to four words, not necessarily grammatical, can be heard.

HEARING: Hearing develops after the first few days of life, but a deaf infant may show no signs of deafness for many months. One of the first things noted in a deaf child is less-than-normal vocalization and not much laughter and smiling. After about one month of age, the child can localize and recognize where noises are coming from. By three months, he can recognize familiar voices, and after six months, may respond to music. If the child is extremely attentive visually, it may be a sign that hearing is not normal. This should be quickly investigated.

TASTE, TOUCH AND SMELL: The sense of taste is present at birth, but it is not known whether the child can differentiate sour, salt, and bitter tastes. By two or three months, taste is sharper and the child can notice a change in the amounts of sugar or other definite tastes in his food. He begins to salivate at about the third month. The lips and tongue of the infant are developed at birth. Localization of touch is developed by the fifth month.

Sense of smell is present in the premature and full-term infant, but this develops slowly. It becomes more acute later on. Most new infants can smell milk.

BURPING: Burping or bubbling the infant is necessary to get rid of gas or air which accumulates in the stomach. If this is not done, the air may cause discomfort, cramps, and mechanical vomiting. The latter is readily seen when the child brings up a great deal of food along with a large amount of gas. In these cases, it may be necessary to burp the baby before and frequently during a feeding, as well as afterwards.

JAUNDICE: This is a yellow discoloration of the skin and eyes produced when red blood cells disintegrate: they release hemoglobin which is changed to bilirubin (a bile pigment). This causes the yellow color.

Physiologic jaundice occurs during the first few days of life. There is increased destruction of red blood cells and decreased excretion of the bile pigment by the infant's immature liver. This type of jaundice usually appears from the second to the fourth day and may disappear by the seventh or fourteenth day. Such jaundice is perfectly normal and is seen in about 40 per cent of all newborn infants. There is no associated enlargement of the liver or spleen and the blood tests are normal in this condition.

PREMATURE BABIES: An infant who weighs five and a half pounds or less is termed premature. This definition applies, whether the child is born at the full term or earlier. Children who are born before term usually weigh less than normal and therefore, automatically, are called premature ("premies").

MORNING SICKNESS: Many pregnant women experience nausea of varying degrees during the first third of their pregnancies. There is no doubt that some physical change in the digestive tract is responsible for this complaint. Worries and anxieties about pregnancy may increase complaints regarding nausea, much as tension may increase a headache or stomach cramps. In addition, anything that can produce or contribute to nausea in the non-pregnant state will do the same to a pregnant woman—whether it be an unpleasant sight or thought, greasy food, or unpleasant odors. Both physical and psychological factors may contribute to morning sickness.

BABY BLUES or post-partum depression is a common term used to describe the depression that many women experience soon after labor and delivery. It has been estimated that at least 60 per cent, and probably more, of new mothers experience definite depression during the first week after delivery. Some women are ashamed to admit this and are puzzled by it. Various emotionally-tinged thoughts occur to the new mother. She may feel that having at long last fulfilled her biological role and becoming a mother is a frightening experience. She may also have doubts and fears about the responsibilities of motherhood and the day-in, day-out commitments this represents. "Baby blues" are widespread in every maternity hospital; they are generally quite temporary and tend to disappear when the mother goes home with her new baby. There is certainly no need, nor is it advisable, to conceal her feelings. She should by all means discuss them with her husband and her doctor.

INTERTRIGO: This is a chafing from the effects of heat and moisture, and is seen in the creases of the infant's skin, particularly in fat babies. It usually occurs in the groin, neck and underneath the armpits. Proper cleansing and proper washing of the skin, as well as changing soiled diapers frequently, is important in the prevention of this condition.

ROSEOLA: Convulsions frequently usher in roseola with high fever up to 105° and 106°F. There is little to explain the sudden onset and marked irritability in this condition except, sometimes, a slight sore throat. The fever remains high and fluctuating for three or four days;

then it suddenly drops and a rash breaks out, usually on the trunk, subsequently spreading to the arms and neck, occasionally on the face. The rash is light pink, flat, approximately the size of peas. It fades within twenty-four to forty-eight hours. A doctor should be consulted if it persists.

RHEUMATIC FEVER: Rheumatic fever is caused by the toxic effect of streptococcus infections in children. These tonsillitis and strep throat infections occur more commonly in the spring in the eastern United States, and on the west coast during the winter. The disease may run in families and is most common where there is poverty, malnutrition, and poor hygiene. Rheumatic fever treatment consists of bed rest, antibiotics, sometimes steroids (cortisone). All children who have had rheumatic fever should be placed on preventative treatment with antibiotics to prevent future infections.

URTICARIA (HIVES): Hives are small, red, raised lesions of the skin which appear suddenly and cause severe itching. They may appear as single pimples or in clusters, and may be large in diameter or very tiny.

Giant hives are characterized by large areas of swelling (edema) which may appear in any part of the skin or mucous membranes. There may be swelling and puffiness of the eyes and lids, and swelling of the throat in which there may be a sensation of choking. The skin may become red and itchy. The causes are generally the same as those of hives; that is, some allergen or possibly a psychological reason. The treatment is the same as for other allergies.

IMPETIGO: This is a contagious disease of the skin characterized by pustules and crusts. It is a common secondary result of any irritation or rash; and appears most commonly on the face, hands, neck, ears, and upper and lower extremities. It starts as a pimple which becomes a blister, filling with pus. Then the yellowish material drains out and produces a raw, wet, pustular surface. Treatment is with antibiotics, either in ointment form or by injection.

STEAM: Steam inhalations are often prescribed when children have croup, hoarseness, sore throat, or difficulty in breathing. Inhaling a warm, moist mixture of air usually relieves the swelling in the tissues of the nose and throat and eases breathing. There are many good commercial vaporizers available. If you buy one, it is important to get the type which will run automatically all night so that you do not have to get up to replace the water.

SUNBURN: The sun's rays can produce injury to the skin comparable to that caused by a flame. One of the differences is that in sunburn, the extent of the injury may be detected only after some hours, and its development is gradual. In addition to reddening and burning sensations, blistering may occur. When a considerable skin area is involved, the person may feel sick and have chilly sensations, weakness, and perhaps also headache and some fever. In most instances sunburn is due to an over-enthusiastic attempt to become tanned too rapidly. Infants and children are very susceptible.

Numerous commercial preparations are available for screening out the skin-damaging components of sunshine. Discomfort can be relieved by powders containing zinc oxide and zinc stearate, or by local applications of calamine lotion, cold cream or special burn preparations. Your doctor can recommend the best types.

TEMPER TANTRUMS: Temper tantrums are characterized by screaming, kicking, breath-holding, and extreme agitation. These are a device often used by infants or children when they are frustrated or refused something they want. They may become angry or jealous, and may use this method to blackmail parents into giving in to them. It is a fairly common behavior reaction in children from one to four. If a temper tantrum is met with indifference, the child will soon observed that kicking and screaming serves no good purpose and is self-defeating. If a child is given what he wishes because parents become intimidated, he will learn that he can do this whenever he wishes to get his way. It is a very bad emotional habit to encourage. It is not usually necessary to punish the child who has temper tantrums. Just refusing to recognize them and handling the situation with calm and firm tolerance is best.

TETANUS (LOCKJAW): This is caused by a contaminated wound. The organism causing this disease is widely distributed in the soil in many parts of the world. Under certain conditions, it gets into the skin and bloodstream and produces several poisons. One of these destroys red blood cells, another injures white blood cells and produces a poison which causes the muscle rigidity and spasm for which this disease is famous. There is no suitable skin test to determine immunity. Any type of wound may give rise to tetanus if the germs enter that area; any injury or skin cut which has been contaminated by dirt should therefore be carefully cleansed and treated, and immunization given to prevent tetanus.

THUMBSUCKING: Sucking is a reflex activity in newborn infants. It is one of the child's first pleasures and satisfactions. Unless adequate sucking is given to children, many develop unsatisfied "oral" needs. Some babies finish the bottle rapidly, not really getting enough sucking. They may continue to suck on their thumbs or fingers because it is pleasurable. Pacifiers replace fingers with some infants. Sucking needs usually diminish after the children are able to drink from a cup or glass, but many of them continue to suck their thumbs for years afterwards. However, most cases of finger- or thumb-sucking are outgrown after the age of two or so, when the child is able to move about on his own and is not entirely dependent upon parents for the satisfactions of needs. Most children who feel a firm family affection and receive sufficient attention do not need to resort to thumb-sucking.

WHOOPING COUGH (PERTUSSIS): This disease occurs most commonly in January and February in northern climates and in May in southern climates. It may occur at any age but is particularly serious if it occurs in infants below one year of age. Active immunization of all infants should be started by the third month of age. This consists of a quadruple injection (diphtheria, pertussis, tetanus, polio) vaccine. It is usually given in monthly injections for three months, followed by booster doses at one year of age and every three years thereafter.

TEETHING: This is a natural phenomenon. Every baby teethes, and between the ages of about five months and two years, it is a fairly constant process. Teething does not cause illness. It is true that the gum over an erupting tooth can become irritated and cause varying degrees of discomfort, as evidenced by increased fussiness and irritability. It should be possible in these instances to use some reliable means to relieve the pain of the swollen gum. If a baby fusses and cries continually, it might possibly cause a slight elevation of temperature. Teeth erupt in the following order: First, the two lower front incisors. The upper two, or four, are next to appear. The average quota is about six teeth around the end of the first year. In the second year, about ten more teeth usually appear—the two lower incisors, the first molars and the canines, or eye teeth. The last teeth to appear are the second molars, at about two years of age or over. They are called deciduous since they will begin to fall out, one by one, to be replaced by permanent teeth at five or six years of age.

INDEX

A

Abortion, 34, 35
Abdominal examination, 42, 44
Abdominal Pains
  in pregnancy, 26
  in colic, 77, 78
Abnormality in pregnancy, 34
Abrasions, 65
Ace bandage, 28
Accepting the new baby, 162-167
Accidents, 83, 208, 218
Adenoids, 94
Adjusting
  to new baby, 55, 59, 69
  to family, 80-84
Advances in pregnancy, 34
Aggressiveness in children, 189-194
Air bubble, 70, 71, 132
Airings, 52, 57, 59, 62, 215
Airplane travel when pregnant, 36
Alcohol in cleansing, 69
Alcoholic beverages
  in pregnancy, 38
  after childbirth, 53
Allergy, 157-160
  what it is, 157-160
  signs of, 158, 159
  history of, 158, 159
  detecting, 159
Allergies, food, 151, 156, 214
  eggs, 133, 151, 152

meats, 152
milk, 76, 77, 151
fruit juice, 154
green pepper, 151
uriticaria, 64
wheat, 151, 154
Allergies, others, 100, 157–160, 212, 214
  animals, 160
  asthma, 157, 158
  dust, 157
  drugs, 64, 157, 160
  eczema, 158
  feathers, 157
  household chemicals, 157
  insects, 157
  mold, 157
  perfume, 157
  pollen, 157
Ambidexterity, 202
American Academy of Allergy, 157
American Dietetic Association, 155
Ammonia in diapers, 60, 61
Anemia
  in pregnancy, 44
  in infancy, 21, 46, 98
  in Rh, 45
Anesthesia, 32, 57
Anger
  in children, 189
  temper tantrums, 168, 169, 189, 227
Animals, nutrition studies, 21, 22
Animal bites, 219

fears of, 204
Ankles, weakness in, 117, 118
Anti-acids, 25, 29
Antibiotics, 64, 65, 98, 212
Antibodies
  against disease, 220
  against Rh, 45, 46
Antihistamine, 29, 99
Antiseptics in diaper washing, 61, 65
Antitoxin, 65
Anxieties in children, 201
A.P.C. Virus, 94
Appetite
  in pregnancy, 17
  loss of, 98, 149
Apples, 18, 26
Applesauce, 133, 142
Arguing with children, 189
Ascorbic acid, 127
Asparagus, 16
Aspirin, 99, 214, 217
Asthma, 157–158
Attention, demand for, 164, 180, 192
Attitudes toward food, 149
Automobile travel, 35, 36, 53
A Vitamins, 16, 17, 72, 126, 127, 148
Awareness in infants, 184

B

Baby blues, 50, 51, 55, 56, 69, 225

INDEX

Baby food
 starting, 131, 135
 adding new foods, 131, 135, 145
 junior foods, 143-144
Baby powder, oil, cream, 62, 63, 65, 67, 69
Baby sitter, 218, 219
Back, supporting, 67
Bacon, 129, 133, 141
Bacteria, 60, 93
Bad habits, 80, 83, 172, 175
Bananas, 133, 142, 153
Bandages, 28
Barefoot walking, 40, 41, 118
Barley, 17
Bathing
 after childbirth, 51, 53
 the baby, 68, 69, 169
Beans
 green, 16
 lima, 16
Bedding, 57
Bedtime (see Sleep)
Bedwetting, 106, 168
Bee stings, 219
Beef, 16, 17
Beets, 142
Behavior patterns, 58, 59, 81, 83, 170
Between-meal snacks, 149, 154
Bicarbonate of soda, 25, 219
Birth defects, 19
Birthday parties, 149
Bites
 animal, 219
 insect, 219
Bladder training, 106
Blankets, 67
Bleeding, 44, 50, 220
Blisters, 60
Blocking in speech, 200-203
Blood tests
 for Rh, 45
 for PKU, 88
 transfusions, 45
Blotchy skin in infants, 63
Boiling diapers, 61
Booties, 117
Boric acid, 65
Bottle feeding
 refusal, 58
 schedules, 170
 bubbling, 58, 71, 224
 formulas, 70
 spitting up, 71, 214
 nipples, 57, 58, 70, 71
 prepared formula, 70, 71, 129
 propping bottles, 70, 127
 weaning, 131, 136
 without sterilization, 129
Bowel movements
 diarrhea, 214, 215
 constipation, 25, 213
 changes in infancy, 64, 72, 74
 enemas, 27, 77
 looseness, 72
 suppositories, 27
 number, 72
Bowel training, 82, 106
 readiness for, 84, 106, 107

INDEX

parents' attitude, 83, 84
resistance, 109, 110
types of seat, 106, 107
schedule, 84
Bowlegs, 116
Brain damage
in Rh, 46
from PKU, 88
Bread
in pregnancy diet, 17
in childhood, 147, 153
non-allergenic, 154
Bread-and-butter snack, 18
Breast feeding, 55, 125, 126, 135
mother's diet, 53
problems, 56, 65
weaning, 136
British Guiana, 48
Broccoli, 16
Bronchitis, 94, 99, 157
Bruises, 216
Brussels sprouts, 16
Bullying, 191
Burns, 216
Burping (bubbling), 56, 58, 71, 78, 132, 224
Butter, 17, 148
Buttermilk, 16
B Vitamins, 16, 148, 153

C

Cabbage, 16
Cakes, cookies, 24, 151, 154
Calamine lotion, 219
Calcium, 145, 146, 153, 219
Calories
in pregnancy diet, 15, 17
in childhood, 146, 148, 151
Calluses, 39
Candy, 149, 151
Canteloupe, 153
Carbohydrates, 15, 17, 24
Carrots, 16
Cavities (caries), 32
Cereals, 17, 26, 129, 132, 137, 147
Cervix, 44
Chafing—chapping, 64, 65
Chard, Swiss, 16
Cheating, 175
Cheese, 16, 147, 153
Cherries, 149
Chewing gum, 25
Chicago Dietetic Supply House, 155
Chicken pox, 210
Childbirth, natural, 50
Chilling, 98
Chloral, 65
Chopped foods, 133
Chubby baby, 64, 144
Circumcision, 57, 60, 61, 69, 221
Citrus fruits, 16, 127, 132, 148, 153
Cleanliness, 172, 193
Cleft palate, 19
Clothing, 57, 59, 76, 81, 192
Cocoa, 23
Cod liver oil, 140
Coffee, 17, 23

Cola drinks, 24
Colds, 93, 212
  causes, 93, 94, 97, 98
  care of, 97-101
  fever, 98, 99
  vaporizer, 99
  enlarged glands, 100
  antibiotics, 99, 100
  respiratory infections, 93, 94, 97
Colic, 58, 76, 82, 212
Collections in childhood, 192
Competition for attention, 163, 189
Compazine, 24
Complications of pregnancy, 34
Condiments, 17
Conduct, rules of, 172, 173
Confidence in child, 192
Conforming in infancy, 172
Conjunctivitis, 94
Constipation, 25, 213
Contractions, 50
Contrariness, 172, 180, 189
Convalescence after childbirth, 52
Convulsions, 88, 220
Coordination, 114
Cord, umbilical, 57, 69, 217
Corn, 142
Corn meal, 17
Corn syrup, 149
Corns (also calluses, warts), 39

Cough
  in colds, 97, 100
  in allergies, 157, 215
  in other illnesses, 100, 215
  care of, 97, 98
Couvade, 48
Coxsacki virus, 94
Crackers, 18, 23, 24
Cradle cap, 212, 215
Creeping, 102, 114
Crib, 70, 74, 163
  for premies, 85
Crossed eyes, 57
Croup, 94, 212
Crying
  in newborn, 56, 69, 74, 80, 81, 168
  at bedtime, 74
  ready to sleep, 74
  ready to play, 70
  in colic, 76
  from hunger, 70, 131, 168
  from wet diaper, 69
  crankiness, 74
  hypertonic baby, 79
  from spoiling, 58, 176, 196
  from discomfort, 69, 70, 168
Cucumbers, 153
Cuddling the baby, 58, 59, 68, 78
Cup for weaning, 136
  for drinking, 136
Custard, 133, 141
Cuts, 65, 216
C Vitamins, 16, 72, 127, 132, 148, 153

INDEX

Cycles in child care, 80

D

Daily schedule, 66, 80, 135
Dancing in pregnancy, 35
Dark, fear of, 181, 206
Dates, 26
Dawdling on potty, 109, 110
 over meals, 150
Decay, dental, 31
Deceitfulness, 175
Defying parents, 166
Delivery of baby, 50, 51
"Demand" feeding, 80
Denis Brown Bar, 116
Dental care in pregnancy, 30-33
Dependency in childhood, 173, 177, 187, 199
Depression
 after childbirth, 50, 51, 55, 56, 69, 225
Depriving the child, 182
Desserts, 49
Destructiveness, 191
Development of child
 in infancy, 102-104
 in toddlerhood, 102-104, 145
 physical growth, 145-150
 personality, 168, 184
 talking, 200
 walking, 103, 147
 habits, 172-179
 seeing, 102, 103

Diapers, 51, 60, 61, 64, 81
Diaper rash, 60-62, 63, 65, 67
Diaper service, 61
Diarrhea, 214, 215
Diet (also see Foods)
 deficiency, 19, 20, 21, 63
 for expectant mother, 14-18, 19, 21, 31, 44, 49
 for infant, 64
 for older child, 145-149
 for father, 49
 nursing mother, 53
 supplements in pregnancy, 15, 16
 in PKU, 91
Dietary supplements, 16
Dietitians, 152, 155
Diphtheria, 65, 96, 97
Discipline, 80, 174, 178, 180, 202
Diseases, 93, 122, 210
Disobedience, 83, 162-164, 168, 175
Disposable bottles, 71, 129
Distracting the child, 166, 182
District Dietetic Ass'n., 155
Diuretic, 14, 15
Doctor, visits to, 44, 53, 79, 91
Douching, 53
Drinking from cup, 136
Drinking alcohol in pregnancy, 38

Driving during pregnancy, 36, 53
Driving after childbirth, 53
Drugs, 64
  for allergy, 160
Dust in allergy, 160
D Vitamins, 72, 127, 132, 147

E

Early training, 106, 172
Ears
  earache, 94, 100, 213
  infections, 94, 95, 100
Eating
  in pregnancy, 14-18, 24
  refusal to, 148, 149
  new foods, 131
  habits, 145-150
  table foods, 131
  between meals, 149
  with family, 131
Echo virus, 94
Eczema, 64, 88, 158
Edema, 43, 44, 64
Eggs
  in pregnancy diet, 16, 17, 23
  in infancy, 129, 134, 140, 141, 147
  allergy to, 133, 151, 152
Elastic stockings, 28, 40
Electrocardiogram, fetal, 43
Embryo, 20
Emotional instability, 168, 170, 184, 190
Emptying breasts, 136
Endive, 16
Enemas, 27, 77
Energetic child, 193, 194
Enriched breads, 17
Enuresis, 111, 168
Environment, influences, 20, 184-187, 189
Enzymes in PKU, 88
Eruptions, skin, 63, 65
Erysibelas, 64
Erythema, 64
Erythroblastosis (Rh), 45-47
E Vitamin, 22
Examination for twins, 44
Examination of new mother, 53
Exchange transfusions, 45
Exercise
  in pregnancy, 26, 34, 35
  for feet, 40, 119
Exotic foods in baby's diet, 142
Expectant parents' classes, 49
Extra foods, 148, 149, 151
Eyes
  in newborn, 55, 63
  baby's sight, 113
  coordination of hands and eyes, 114
  vision examination, 115
  crossed eyes, 57
  conjunctivitis, 94
  strabismus, 57

INDEX

F

Falls, 116
Family
  baby adapting to, 142, 143
  management of problems, 162, 168, 172, 180
  disorganized family, 201
Fat
  in diet, 15
  in infancy, 63
  in milk, 63
Father
  role in pregnancy, 48-51
  in the delivery room, 50, 51
  role in discipline, 180
  adjustment to baby, 51, 127
Fatigue
  in pregnancy, 35, 36
  in motherhood, 66, 76
Favoritism, 162
Fear of dentistry, 32
Fears, 204-208
  about handling baby, 69
  infancy, 168, 170, 204
  parental influence, 170, 205
  of animals, 205, 206
  of the dark, 181
  of lightning, 205
  of strangers, 170, 171, 195
  of water, 204
Feedings
  individual baby's needs, 55, 56, 70, 73
  bottle feeding, 58, 70, 125, 126
  breast feeding, 56, 58, 125, 126
  in the hospital, 55, 70, 125
  first days at home, 56, 57, 70, 73
  refusal, 56, 58, 81, 82
  making a schedule, 83
  self-regulating, 81, 128
  without warming, 129, 130
  night feedings, 73, 74
  feeding the premie, 86
  first solids, 58, 81, 82, 129
  combination feedings, 130, 135
  meats, 129
  introducing new foods, 58, 79, 82, 145
  three meals a day, 129, 149
  trends in feeding, 130
Feeding problems
  colic, 76
  smaller appetite, 143, 145
  refusal of new foods, 82, 128, 141, 145
  refusal to eat, 56, 82, 145, 149
  preference for sweets, 58, 141, 148, 149
  after illness, 98
  learning to feed himself, 145, 150

INDEX

Feeding problems (Cont.)
  dawdling at meals, 150
  mother's urging, 58, 82, 83, 149
  spitting up, 71
Feelings
  about the baby, 55, 69
  after delivery, 55, 56
  baby blues, 50, 51, 56
Feet
  care of in pregnancy, 39, 40, 41
  in infancy, 116
  flat feet, 116
  walking, 116
  types of shoes, 39, 116
  exercises for, 40, 41, 119
Fetal heartbeat, 43
Fetus, 19, 20, 36, 37
Fever (see colds), 98, 100, 214, 217
  how to reduce, 214
Figs, 26
Finger sucking, 84
First aid
  bites, 219
  bleeding, 44, 50, 220
  burns, 216
  convulsions, 220
  cuts, 216
  nosebleeds, 216
  skin infections, 60, 63, 215
  stings, 219
First baby, 106
First steps, 117
First-time mother, 55-59, 66, 69, 106
First walker, 117
Fish
  in pregnancy diet, 16, 17
  in children's diet, 147
Fitting shoes
  in infancy, 117
  in pregnancy, 39
Flat feet, 116
Flexibility, 83, 106
Fluids, 17, 24, 26, 99
Food Groups, 152
Foods
  pregnancy diet, 14-18, 25, 44
  in infancy, 79, 129
  for morning sickness, 23, 25
  for nursing mother, 125, 126
  introducing new foods, 58, 130, 145
  family foods, 142, 145
  variations in texture, 58
  impacted in teeth, 31
Formulas, 57, 70, 79, 125-129 (see also bottle feeding)
Fortified milk, 16
Fragility, 59
Fresh air, 24, 57, 59, 215
Fried foods, 25
Frightening the child, 204
Frostings, 149
Fruits, 26, 58, 110, 133, 148
Fruit juice, 16, 17, 23, 26, 139

Frustration in childhood, 79, 81, 82, 174, 190

G

Gagging, 141
Gaining weight
  in pregnancy, 14, 15, 43, 44
  in childhood, 145
Gamma globulin, 46, 47
Garter belt, 28
Gas
  in dentistry, 32
  in stomach, 70, 71, 76, 77
Genes, 221
Genetic defect, 88
Gentian violet, 56
German measles (rubella), 65
Germs, 99
Getting attention, 179, 180
Getting his way, 172, 180, 191
Gingerale, 24
Gingivitis, 30, 31
Girdle, 28, 53
Giving in to child, 80-84
Glands, enlarged, 100
Gnat bites, 219
Good habits, 173
  formation of, 176
Golf
  during pregnancy, 35
Graham crackers, 24
Grams in food, 147
Grandparents, 76, 103, 115
Grapefruit, 153

Grapes, 149
Great Britain, studies in, 21
Green beans, 16
Green peppers, 16, 17, 152, 153
Green vegetables, 148, 153
Greens, salad, 16, 152
Growing child, 84, 145, 166, 167
Growth rate
  of fetus, 15
  of baby, 145
  of toddler, 145
Gums, 30
Gunthire test for PKU, 91

H

Habits
  good and bad, 82, 172
  in eating, 149
Hair of newborn, 57
Handedness, shift of, 202
Hand-eye coordination, 114
Hand-me-down shoes, 117
Hands
  in infancy, 102
  how babies use, 102
Harvard School of Public Health nutrition studies, 21
Hay fever, 157
Hazardous foods
  for toddlers, 148, 149
Head
  in infancy, 55, 59, 67
Health record, 210, 211

Hearing, 56, 102, 223
Heartburn, 25, 221
Heat rash, 57, 58, 63
Help at home, 66, 69
Hemorrhoids, 53, 222
Hemoglobin, 21
Heredity, 20, 22, 27, 64, 88, 145, 184, 181
Hiccups, 57
High blood pressure, 14, 44
High shoes for babies, 117
High strung babies, 78, 79, 185, 205
Hiking in pregnancy, 35
Hitting, 189
Hives, 64, 226
Holding the baby, 59, 67, 131
Holland, nutrition during war, 20
Home care of premature baby, 87
Homecoming with baby, 55, 56, 69, 80
Honey, 23
Hormonal changes in pregnancy, 30, 55
Horseback riding
  in pregnancy, 35
Hospital
  care for baby, 56
  premature baby, 85
  feeding practices, 125, 137
  father in delivery room, 50, 51
  for twins, 44
Hostility in childhood, 168, 180, 189
Hot water bottle, 77
House dust in allergies, 157
Humor, sense of, 165
Hunger cry, 70
Hurting other children, 175
Husbands
  during pregnancy, 48
  in delivery room, 50, 51
Hypertonic baby, 78
Hypnotics, 37

I

Ice cream, 16, 23, 24
Indigestion in pregnancy, 25
  in babies, 76
Infections, 62, 65, 98, 99
Illnesses
  of baby, 97
  of toddler, 98, 190
  in family, 93
  care of sick baby, 95, 97
  colds, 93, 95, 97-101
  rashes, 160, 162
  diseases, 93
  fever, 95, 100
  giving medicine, 95
  vaporizer, 99
Immunity, of baby, 86, 94, 97, 126, 135
Immunizations, 93, 97, 122, 210, 211, 222
  for allergy, 160

INDEX

Impactions, food, 31
Impetigo, 226
Inadequacy in childhood, 190
Incubator for premies, 85
Independence
  at mealtime, 135, 145
Indigestion
  in pregnancy, 25
  in infancy, 69, 76
Individuality in babies, 74, 76, 131
Infant mortality, 19, 45, 46
Infantile paralysis, 122, 210 (poliomyelitis)
Infections, prevention of, 85, 86, 93, 99, 100
Ingrown nails, 116
Injuries
  cuts, 65, 216
  burns, 216
  nose and throat, 97
  prevention of, 218
Inoculations
  diphtheria, 65, 95, 122
  D.P.T., 122
  lockjaw (tetanus), 122
  measles, 195
  pertussis (whooping cough), 122, 229
  poliomyelitis, 122
  tuberculin test, 122
Insect bites, 157, 219
Instability, emotional, 168
Intelligence, 184
Intestines, 60
Intestinal upsets, 26
  colic, 76, 212
  diarrhea, 214, 215
  in heartburn, 26
  hiccups, 57
  spitting up, 71, 214
  vomiting, 198, 214
Institute of Human Potential, 102, 104
Intercourse, 53
Intertrigo, 225
Intradermal test for allergy, 159
Intussusception, 222
Iodides, 65
Iodine, 216
I.Q., 221
Iron
  in pregnancy diet, 16, 21, 44, 127
  deficiency, 21
  in childhood, 148, 153
Itching, 64, 157

J

Jams, jellies, 18, 23, 149
  marmalade, 23
Jaundice, 46, 56, 224
Jealousy
  when baby comes home, 163, 164
  sibling jealousy, 161-167
Juices, fruit, 16, 17, 23 (canned, frozen or fresh)
Junior foods, 142

K

Kale, 16, 153
Kicking, 169, 182
Kidneys, 15, 64
Kindergarten, 195
Knock knees, 116

L

Labor, 35, 44, 50, 55
Labority test for twins, 43
Lamp in baby's room, 113
Language (speech development), 200, 223
Lanolin, 65
Laundry service for diapers, 60, 61
Laxatives, 27
Laziness
 in toilet training, 106
Leadership, 192
Leafy vegetables, 14, 148
Learning
 to swallow, 131
 to drink from cup, 136
 to feed himself, 150
 to talk, 223
 to walk, 116
 in first year, 172
Left-and-right-handedness, 202
Leg cramps, 28
Legs, development of, 120
Lemon juice, 24
Leningrad, diet in wartime, 20, 21
Lettuce, leaf, 16
Licorice, 26
Liquids, 26
Liver, 16, 17, 148, 153
Lockjaw (tetanus), 228
Loneliness in childhood, 80, 169, 195
Lotion, baby, 63, 69
Love from parents, 66, 181, 186, 201
Low shoes in babyhood, 119
Lying, 172

M

Magnesia tablets, 25
Malformations in infancy, 19, 20
Malnutrition, 20, 21
Malted milk, 24
Management of pregnancy, 14, 23, 30, 34
Management of twin pregnancy, 42-44
Managing toddlers
 aggressiveness, 189
 balkiness, 180
 bedtime, 73
 dawdling, 109, 150
 discipline, 180
 distracting, 166, 182
 father's role, 180
 fears, 206, 207
 naps, 73
 outgoingness, 180, 195, 198
 play, 98, 114, 189, 197

problem behavior, 169, 170
tantrums, 169, 170, 189
timidity, 195
toileting, 106-112
toys, 114, 115, 148
training, 172, 180
Margarine, fortified, 17, 148
Marital relations, 50, 53
Masks with premies, 86
Massage, 28, 29
Masturbation, 175
Matriarchy, 48
Meals
  in pregnancy, 17, 18, 23, 24, 25
  in infancy, 58, 129
  in toddlerhood, 129, 145-150
  three-a-day, 17, 18, 129
  between-meal snacks, 149
Measles, 95, 97, 122-123
  in pregnancy, 23-24
Meat
  in pregnancy diet, 16, 17, 23, 24
  in baby's diet, 58, 129, 133, 138, 147
  scraped meat, 133
Meningitis, 69, 95
Menstrual periods, 50
Mental retardation, 88-91
Menus for allergies, 152
Middle child, 191
Midnight feedings, doing away with, 139

Midwives, 34
Milk
  breast, 126, 127
  in pregnancy diet, 16, 17, 18, 23, 24
  from a cup, 136
  fortified, 132
  prepared formula, 129
  skimmed, 14-18
  refusal of, 145
  in nursing mother's diet, 53, 126
  baby's need for, 73, 125, 131, 147, 153
Milk, mother's, 125-129
Milk of magnesia, 25, 27
Mineral oil, 26, 27
Minerals in diet, 15, 17, 227
Miscarriage, 19, 34, 35, 47
Mobile in baby's room, 113
Momism, 202
Monilia (thrush), 56, 60
Morning sickness, 23, 225
Moro reflex, 204
Mortality, newborn, 19, 45, 46
Mosquito bites, 219
Motherhood, 59, 66, 69, 186
Motoring in pregnancy, 35
Motion sickness, 35, 36
Mouth care
  thrush, 56, 60
Mucus, 98, 99
Multiple births, 41-43, 217
Mumps, 211

Muscles
  in feet and legs, 39, 40, 89, 114
  growth of, 145, 148
Muscle cramps, 28, 29

N

Nagging child, 181
Nails, 39, 40
Nail biting, 175
Naps
  in pregnancy, 38, 44
  in infancy, 73
  after childbirth, 52
National Jewish Hospital, Denver, 158, 160
Natural childbirth, 50, 51
Nausea (morning sickness), 23, 24, 49, 224
Navel, 42, 69, 217
Neatness, 172
Neck muscles, 67
Negativism in child, 166
Nervous baby, 78
Nervous system in infancy, 79, 205
Nervousness
  in mothers, 74, 79
  in infancy, 77, 78, 205
  fears, 203, 204
New baby at home, 56, 87, 163, 164
Newborn traits, 55-59, 69-72, 73, 87, 184
Niacin, 126, 127
Night feedings, 83, 139

Nightmares, 168, 169
Nipples
  on bottles, 58, 70
  nursing mother's, 56
  size of holes, 58, 77, 78
"No" phase, 164, 165, 167, 173
Non-allergenic foods & menus, 151
Non-fat dry milk, 136
Normal development, 142-143
Nose
  allergies, 157
  bleeding, 216
  in colds, 98
Nose picking, 175
Novocaine, 32
Nurse
  in hospital, 56
  visiting, 87
Nursery care of premies, 87
Nursery furniture, 76
Nursery, hospital, 85
Nursery school, 198
Nutritional requirements
  before childbirth, 19, 20, 31, 125
  nursing mother, 56
  infant and toddler, 97, 149, 152
  in prematures, 85, 87
Nuts, 149

O

Oatmeal, 23, 26

INDEX

Obedience, 176, 179
Obesity, 15
Obstetrician, 14-18, 34, 35, 47, 48, 55
Oil
  baby oil, 62, 63
  mineral oil, 26, 27
  in dressing, 23
Old wives' tales, 30
Older child, 162, 163, 190
One year old child
  dependence, 83, 84, 145
  development, 79, 102, 145
  exploring, 102
  fears, 168, 195, 205
  habits, 80, 84, 145
  loss of appetite, 143, 144, 145
  managing him, 82, 83, 168, 189
  personality, 79, 102, 145, 184
  playing, 102
  sleep, 73-75, 83, 84, 168, 175
  temper tantrums, 168, 189
  toilet training, 82, 83, 168
  variations in appetite, 83, 84, 145
Orange juice, 24
Outgoing child, 180, 195, 198
Outings, 57, 59, 215
Overeating, 14
Over-discipline, 84, 189, 195
Over-indulgence, 190
Over-protection of child, 168, 195
Overweight child, 149
Oxfords, 39, 119
Oxide, zinc, 65
Oxygen, 36, 87, 212
Oysters, 17

P

Pacifiers, 170, 171, 228
Pain, feelings of
  in infancy, 56, 57, 65, 95, 187
  in colic, 76, 77, 78, 212
  with disease, 89, 93-96, 100
Pampering, 168, 176
Parents
  adjustment to parenthood, 55, 69, 80, 131, 164
  caring for baby, 55, 60, 63, 69, 73, 80
  disciplining child, 168, 169, 189
  feelings about children, 163
  problems of, 190, 196
  self-confidence, 66, 69, 73, 131, 134, 175
  spoiling, 165, 189, 190
  worries of, 163, 164, 168, 175, 176, 189

Parties, 193
Passive transfer test for allergies, 159
Patience with children, 79, 173, 175, 208
Peaches, 142
Pears, 142
Peas, 16
Pediatrician, 55, 56, 59, 63, 65, 69, 81, 105, 119
Pelvis, 43
Penis, 60, 69
Peppers, green, 17
Permissiveness, 80, 180
Personality development, 74, 79, 106, 174, 185-189
Pertussis (whooping cough) 64, 229
Petroleum jelly, 68, 69
Pet names, 164
Phenobarbital, 24
Phenolphthalein, 65
Phenylketonouria (PKU), 88-91
Phenylalanine in PKU, 88-91
Phenylpyruvic acid, 88
Phosphorus, 146, 147
Pigeon toes, 116
Pillow, 57
Pituitary glands, 135
Placenta, 45, 46
Play
in babyhood, 81, 114, 148
in childhood, 197
with other children, 98, 114, 189, 193, 197
with toys, 114, 115, 148
when ill, 99
Play groups, 189, 200
Play pen, 74, 103, 114
Playthings, 114, 115, 182
Pneumonia, 93-96, 99
Podiatrist, 40, 118
Poisons, 61
Poliomyelitis, 122, 210, 211
Pollen, 157
Poor appetite, 143
Popularity in children, 192
Postnatal care, 52
Postpartum examination, 53
Posture in pregnancy, 39
Potatoes, 17, 23, 24, 49, 148
Sweet, 142
Potty chair, 107, 109
Poultry, 16, 17, 152
Powder, baby, 63, 215
foot, 40
Powdered milk, 16
Praise of child, 110, 174, 175
Pregnancy
diet, 14-18, 19-22
health in, 34-38
nutrition in, 19
Premature baby, 20, 21, 85-87, 224
Premature labor, 44
Prepared formula, 55, 70, 71, 129
Pretzels, 134
Prickly heat, 64, 215
Problem behavior, 82, 170, 171

Pronation, 116
Propping bottle, 70, 127
Protein
　in diet, 15, 17, 133, 146, 153, 154
　in PKU, 90
　in premies, 86
Prunes, 26, 142
Psychological effects of pregnancy, 34, 55
Puddings, 134, 141
Pumice stone, 140
Pumpkin, 16
Punishment, 81, 177, 178, 180, 183, 187
Pyloric stenosis, 214
Pylorospasm, 214

Q

Quadruple vaccine, 122, 123, 210
Quarantine, 122, 210
Quarreling, 162
Queasy stomach (nausea), 23
Quick cereals, 132, 137, 138

R

Raisins, 26
Rashes
　diaper, 60, 61, 65, 67, 215
　other, 63, 64, 65, 215
Rate of growth
　of child, 145-150
Rattles, 113
Reading
　starting in school, 102, 103
Ready-to-feed formula, 55
Record, health, 210-211
Recovery from delivery, 52
Rectal thermometer, 212
Reflexes, feeding, 132
Refusing to eat, 171
Regurgitation, 56, 58, 168
Rejection of baby, 186, 201
Reproduction, 19, 20
Resenting the new baby, 163-168
Respiratory allergies, 158
Respiratory infections, 93, 97, 212
Rest (in pregnancy), 36, 52
Rh (erythroblastosis), 45-47
Rheumatic fever, 95, 226
Riboflavin, 126, 148, 153
Rice, 23
Right-and-left-handedness, 202
Rigid schedule, 80
Rivalry, sibling, 162-167
Room for baby, 163
Rooming-in, 55
Rooting, 132
Roseola, 59, 225
Routines in baby care, 55, 66, 69, 76, 80
Rubella, German measles, 65
Rules for habit formation, 84, 175, 176, 177

Rules for new mothers, 52, 53
Running, 147
Running away, 178
Runny nose, 97, 98, 214
Rye, 17, 154
Rye bread (recipe for), 154 (non-allergenic)

S

Sabin vaccine, 210, 211
Safety in infancy, 58
Salads, green, 16, 17, 23, 24, 26
Salk vaccine, 210, 211
Salt, 14, 15, 17, 44
Salt substitutes, 17, 44
Scalding, 60
Scales, 15
Scalp care
  cradle cap, 215
  shampooing, 215
Scarletinal eruption, 65
Scarlet fever, 65
Schedules
  self-regulating, 55, 80, 83
  first schedule, 70, 74, 83, 128
  as baby adjusts, 70, 83, 84, 129
Scolding, 110, 187, 196
School, nursery, 198
Scotland, nutrition in, 21
Screaming in colic, 76
  in tantrums, 169

Sea foods, 16, 17, 23, 24
Second baby, 59, 106
Security in the home
  for baby, 68, 80, 83, 188
  for toddler, 170, 197, 208
Sedatives
  in pregnancy, 24
  in infancy, 79
Self-confidence of mother, 59, 66, 111, 176
Self-demand, 80, 128
Selfishness in childhood, 175
Senses, development of
  in infancy, 56, 102, 103, 113, 223
Sensory, motor behavior, 185
Serum, 65
Sex during pregnancy, 50, 53
Shaming the child, 181, 197
Sharing with siblings, 163
Sherbet, 24
Shift of handedness, 202
Shoes
  baby and toddler, 116
  for expectant mothers, 39
Shots for diseases, 122-123, 220
  for allergy, 160
Shyness, 195-199
Sibling rivalry, 162-167, 190
Sick child, 222
Sight at birth, 56, 57
Skimmed milk, 16

INDEX

Skin care
  in babyhood, 63
  allergies, 64, 157
  care of, 63, 67
  chafing, 64
  diaper rash, 60, 62, 215
  discoloration, 55
  eczema, 157
  impetigo, 226
  irritants of premies, 85
  prickly heat, 64, 215
  rash, 60, 61, 62, 63
  thrush, 215
  urticaria (hives), 64, 226
Slapping, 181
Slaw, cabbage, 17
Sleep
  needs in pregnancy, 36, 37, 38
  in infancy, 66, 73, 81, 168
  on stomach, 58, 71
  sleep problems, 73, 81, 168
  number of hours, 73, 168
Smaller appetite, 143, 144
Smallpox
  inoculations, 122, 210, 211
Smell, 223
Smoking in pregnancy, 37, 38, 53
Smothering, 58
Snacks, 149, 154
Sneakers, 119
Sneezing, 57, 215
Soap, baby, 63, 67

Sociability, 74, 83, 184, 193
Socks, 117
Soft drinks, 24
Solid foods in diet, 58, 79, 81, 129, 130, 132, 133, 134, 142, 143
Sore throat, 95
Sounds in infancy, 102, 204
Soups for baby
  combined with meats, 139
  in pregnancy diets, 17, 23
Soy bean milk, 153
Spanking, 181
Speech development, 200, 223
Spinach, 16, 153
Spitting up, 71, 214
Spoiling, 152, 189, 190
Spoon feeding, 132
Sponge baths, 66, 69
Sportsmanship in childhood, 193
Squash, yellow, 16
Stairs, going up and down after pregnancy, 52
Starches in diet, 15, 64
Steam, vaporizer, 99, 227
  tent, 212
Steps, first, 116
Sterility, 19, 22
Sterilizing formula, 125, 136
Stillbirth, 19, 20
Stings, 219
Stitches, 53
Stockings, elastic, 28, 40

Stomach upsets
　in pregnancy, 25, 26
　in babies, 64
Stools
　in pregnancy, 25, 26
　in infancy, 72
Strabismus, 57
Strained foods, 58, 138, 142
Strangers, fear of, 83, 185
Strawberries, 153
Streptococcus germs, 93
Strictness in parents, 80,
　145, 190, 196, 202
String beans, 153
Stuttering, 200-203
Substituting foods in
　allergies, 151
Sucking
　need for, 125, 132, 135,
　　228
　bottle or breast, 135
　thumb or finger, 228
Sugar
　in pregnancy diet, 14
　in formula, 63, 72, 213
　in infancy, 134, 149
Sulfa drugs, 65
Sulking, 182, 183, 195
Sunbaths, 62, 215, 216
Sunburn, 227
Superstitions, 30
Supplements to pregnancy
　diet, 15
Suppositories, 27
Swabs, 69
Swaddling, 67
Sweet potatoes, 142

Sweets, 134, 141, 149
Swimming during
　pregnancy, 35
Syrup, 149

T

Table foods, 131, 135, 145
Talking, 200, 223
Tangerines, 153
Tartar, 31
Tasting (ability at birth),
　56, 57, 223
Tea, 23
Tears of new mother, 56
　of child, 146, 195
Teeth, care of
　in pregnancy, 30, 31, 125
Teething, 229
Temper tantrums, 168, 169,
　189, 227
Temperament, 174, 184,
　185
Temperature
　of baby's bath, 68
　in illness, 65
　reducing fever, 97
　in premies, 85, 87
Tennis during pregnancy,
　35
Tension in mothers, 66, 67,
　74
Terminal sterilization, 129
Tests
　for PKU, 90
　for Rh, 47
　for allergies, 158, 159

INDEX

Tetanus, (lockjaw), 122, 210, 228
Thiamine, 127, 148
Thinning cereal, 133
Threatening the child, 170, 176, 181
Throat infections, 98
Throwing objects, 176, 189
Thrush (monilia), 56, 60
Thumbsucking, 168, 169, 174, 175, 228
Timidity in children, 195-199
Toenails, 40
Toeing in and out, 116
Toilet training, 81, 84, 106-112, 168, 169, 217
   timetable, 111
   type of seat, 109
Tomato juice, 132
Tomatoes, 16, 153
Tonsils, 217
Tonsilitis, 95, 217
Touch, sense of, 102, 223
Toys, 98, 164, 182
Training, behavior, 173
Transfusions in Rh, 45
Traveling during pregnancy, 36
Treatment for colds, 97-101
Tuberculin test, 122, 123, 210
Turnips, 16, 17
Twins, 42
   watching weight with, 44
Two year olds
   independence, 145
   training, 106
   saying no, 145, 146, 165, 174
   aggressiveness, 189, 194
   timidity, 195
   adjusting to new baby, 162, 163
   punishing, 180-183
   temper tantrums, 169, 189, 227

U

Ulcerations of penis, 60
Ultra-violet rays, 216
Umbilical cord, 42, 57, 69, 217
Understanding the child, 79, 84, 187, 195, 208
Urination
   in infancy, 60
   enuresis, 111, 168
Urine training, 106-112
Urticaria (hives), 64, 226
Uterus, 15, 26, 39, 42, 135

V

Vaccines, 46, 95
Vaccinations (see also Inoculations), 122, 123
Vaginal bleeding, 27
   discomfort, 49
Vaporizer, 99
Varicose veins, 27, 28, 40

Vaseline, 50
Vegetables
  in infancy, 58, 129, 138
  in pregnancy diet, 16, 23, 24, 26
Ventilation, 93
Virus, in colds, 97-101
  others, 93, 94
Vision examination, 115
Vision in infancy, 56, 57, 102, 113
Visiting
  other children, 195
Visiting nurse, 87
Visitors, fear of, 170, 171
Vitamins, 227
  in pregnancy, 15, 22, 127
  for Baby, 58, 72, 97, 140, 147
  for nursing mother, 126
Vomiting
  during pregnancy, 23, 25, 49
  in childhood, 198, 214

W

Walkers, shoes, 116-121
Walking, 103, 147
Walking barefoot, 40, 41
Warts, 39, 216
Water
  in pregnancy, 14, 15, 17, 44
  in baby's diet, 71, 72, 77
  between meals, 72, 137

Watercress, 16
Waterproof pants, 60
Waters, breaking, 44
Weaning, 136, 168, 186
Weighing, how to, 15
Weight gain
  in pregnancy, 14, 15, 17, 18, 43, 44
  in babies, 145
  in toddlers, 145-149
  with twins, 43
Weight of premie, 85
Wetting (see also toilet training), 106
Wheat in allergies, 152-155
Wheat bread, 17, 26
Whining, 168, 179, 182
Whooping cough (pertussis), 64, 97, 229
Womb, 44
Wonder drugs, 60, 64, 95
Working mothers, 66
World, baby's, 67
Worries
  of new mothers, 55
  of children, 204
Wounds, 216

X

X rays, abdominal, 44

Y

Yeast, 60
Yellow Jaundice, 224

INDEX

Yellow vegetables, 16, 148, 153
Yolks, egg, 140
Youngest child, 190

Z

Zinc oxide, 65
Zweiback, 23, 24, 133

Crane Publishing Co., Inc.
Publishers of
My Baby Magazine
and
Congratulations
Magazine

MY BABY MAGAZINE . . .
pick up your free copy
at your favorite store

CONGRATULATIONS MAGAZINE . . .
The Original
hospital-distributed
Baby Magazine